Practice Gaps in Dermatology

Editor

MURAD ALAM

DERMATOLOGIC CLINICS

www.derm.theclinics.com

Consulting Editor

BRUCE H. THIERS

July 2016 • Volume 34 • Number 3

ELSEVIER

1600 John F. Kennedy Boulevard • Suite 1800 • Philadelphia, Pennsylvania, 19103-2899

http://www.theclinics.com

DERMATOLOGIC CLINICS Volume 34, Number 3
July 2016 ISSN 0733-8635, ISBN-13: 978-0-323-44844-4

Editor: Jessica McCool
Developmental Editor: Susan Showalter

Dermatologic Clinics (ISSN 0733-8635) is published quarterly by Elsevier Inc., 360 Park Avenue South, New York, NY 10010-1710. Months of publication are January, April, July, and October. Business and editorial offices: 1600 John F. Kennedy Blvd., Suite 1800, Philadelphia, PA 19103-2899. Customer service office: 11830 Westline Drive, St. Louis, MO 63146. Periodicals postage paid at New York, NY, and additional mailing offices. Subscription prices are USD 370.00 per year for US individuals, USD 618.00 per year for US institutions, USD 425.00 per year for Canadian individuals, USD 754.00 per year for Canadian institutions, USD 495.00 per year for international individuals, USD 754.00 per year for international institutions, USD 100.00 per year for US students/residents, and USD 240.00 per year for Canadian and international students/residents. International air speed delivery is included in all *Clinics* subscription prices. All prices are subject to change without notice. **POSTMASTER:** Send address changes to *Dermatologic Clinics*, Elsevier Health Sciences Division, Subscription Customer Service, 3251 Riverport Lane, Maryland Heights, MO 63043. **Customer Service: 1-800-654-2452 (U.S. and Canada); 314-447-8871 (outside U.S. and Canada). Fax: 314-447-8029. E-mail: journalscustomerservice-usa@elsevier.com (for print support); journalsonlinesupport-usa@elsevier.com (for online support).**

Reprints. For copies of 100 or more, of articles in this publication, please contact the Commercial Reprints Department, Elsevier Inc., 360 Park Avenue South, New York, New York 10010-1710. Tel.: 212-633-3874; Fax: 212-633-3820; Email: reprints@elsevier.com.

The *Dermatologic Clinics* is covered in *MEDLINE/PubMed (Index Medicus)*, *Current Contents/Clinical Medicine*, *Excerpta Medica*, *Chemical Abstracts*, and *ISI/BIOMED*.

Contributors

CONSULTING EDITOR

BRUCE H. THIERS, MD
Professor and Chairman, Department of
Dermatology and Dermatologic Surgery,
Medical University of South Carolina,
Charleston, South Carolina

EDITOR

MURAD ALAM, MD, MSCI, MBA
Professor, Departments of Otolaryngology
and Surgery; Vice-Chair, Department of
Dermatology; Chief, Section of Cutaneous
and Aesthetic Surgery; Director, Micrographic
Surgery and Dermatologic Oncology
Fellowship, Northwestern University, Feinberg
School of Medicine, Chicago, Illinois

AUTHORS

MURAD ALAM, MD, MSCI, MBA
Professor, Departments of Otolaryngology
and Surgery; Vice-Chair, Department of
Dermatology; Chief, Section of Cutaneous
and Aesthetic Surgery; Director, Micrographic
Surgery and Dermatologic Oncology
Fellowship, Northwestern University, Feinberg
School of Medicine, Chicago, Illinois

CRISTINA CARRERA, MD, PhD
Dermatology Service, Department of
Medicine, Memorial Sloan Kettering
Cancer Center, New York, New York;
Melanoma Unit, Department of Dermatology,
Hospital Clinic, IDIBAPS, CIBERER, University
of Barcelona, Barcelona, Spain

TODD V. CARTEE, MD
Assistant Professor of Dermatology,
Department of Dermatology, Pennsylvania
State University, Penn State Milton
S. Hershey Medical Center, Hershey,
Pennsylvania

ARMAND B. COGNETTA Jr, MD
Division of Dermatology, Florida State
University College of Medicine, Tallahassee,
Florida

MARIA L. COLAVINCENZO, MD
Department of Dermatology, Northwestern
University Feinberg School of Medicine,
Chicago, Illinois

M. LAURIN COUNCIL, MD
Assistant Professor of Dermatology,
Division of Dermatology, Department of
Internal Medicine, Washington University in
St. Louis, St. Louis, Missouri

NAZANIN EHSANI-CHIMEH, MD
Postdoctoral Fellow, Department of
Dermatology, Stanford University School of
Medicine, Stanford, California

NICOLE M. FETT, MD, MSCE
Department of Dermatology, Center for Health
and Healing, Oregon Health and Science
University, Portland, Oregon

DAVID FIORENTINO, MD, PhD
Department of Dermatology, Stanford University School of Medicine, Redwood City, California

DAVID J. GOLDBERG, MD, JD
Skin Laser and Surgery Specialists of NY and NJ; Department of Dermatology, Mt. Sinai School of Medicine, New York, New York

ARI M. GOLDMINZ, MD
Department of Dermatology, Tufts Medical Center, Boston, Massachusetts

ALICE B. GOTTLIEB, MD, PhD
Chair and Chief of the Department of Dermatology, Tufts Medical Center, Boston, Massachusetts

JACQUELINE E. GREB, BA
Department of Dermatology, Tufts Medical Center, Boston, Massachusetts

ILTEFAT H. HAMZAVI, MD
Department of Dermatology, Henry Ford Hospital, Detroit, Michigan

ANNA Q. HARE, MD
Resident, Department of Dermatology, Oregon Health and Science University, Portland, Oregon

HYOKYOUNG GRACE HONG, PhD
Department of Statistics and Probability, Michigan State University, East Lansing, Michigan

SHELBY HOPP, BS
Carver College of Medicine, University of Iowa, Iowa City, Iowa

IAN A. MAHER, MD
Assistant Professor, Department of Dermatology, Saint Louis University, St. Louis, Missouri

MICHAEL A. MARCHETTI, MD
Dermatology Service, Department of Medicine, Memorial Sloan Kettering Cancer Center, New York, New York

ASHFAQ A. MARGHOOB, MD
Dermatology Service, Department of Medicine, Memorial Sloan Kettering Cancer Center, New York, New York

MARIA L. MARINO, MD
Dermatology Service, Department of Medicine, Memorial Sloan Kettering Cancer Center, New York, New York

M. PETER MARINKOVICH, MD
Associate Professor, Department of Dermatology, Stanford University School of Medicine, Stanford; Attending Physician, Veterans Administration Medical Center, Palo Alto, California

TASNEEM F. MOHAMMAD, MD
Department of Dermatology, Henry Ford Hospital, Detroit, Michigan

CHRISTEN M. MOWAD, MD
Clinical Professor, Temple University School of Medicine; Department of Medicine, Division of Dermatology, Geisinger Medical Center, Danville, Pennsylvania

KEYVAN NOURI, MD
Professor of Dermatology, Otolaryngology, and Opthalmology; Chief, Dermatology Services, Sylvester Comprehensive Cancer Center; Director, Mohs, Dermatology & Laser Surgery; Director of Surgical Training; Louis C. Skinner, Jr., M.D. Endowed Chair in Dermatology, University of Miami Health System; Department of Dermatology and Cutaneous Surgery, University of Miami Miller School of Medicine, Miami, Florida

TYLER L. QUEST, MD
Chief Resident, Department of Dermatology, University of Iowa Hospitals and Clinics, Iowa City, Iowa

PHOEBE RICH, MD
Adjunct Professor, Department of Dermatology, Oregon Health and Science University; Oregon Dermatology Research Center, Portland, Oregon

JULIE V. SCHAFFER, MD
Division of Pediatric Dermatology, Hackensack University Medical Center, Hackensack, New Jersey

JONATHAN I. SILVERBERG, MD, PhD, MPH
Assistant Professor, Departments of
Dermatology, Preventive Medicine, and
Medical Social Sciences, Northwestern
University Feinberg School of Medicine;
Director, Northwestern Medicine
Multidisciplinary Eczema Center, Chicago,
Illinois

JOSEPH F. SOBANKO, MD
Director, Dermatologic Surgery Education;
Assistant Professor of Dermatology,
Department of Dermatology, University
of Pennsylvania, Philadelphia,
Pennsylvania

ABIGAIL WALDMAN, MD
Fellow, Micrographic Surgery and
Dermatology Oncology, Department of
Dermatology, Northwestern University
Feinberg School of Medicine, Chicago,
Illinois

KAROLYN A. WANAT, MD
Assistant Professor, Departments of
Dermatology, Pathology, and Infectious
Disease, University of Iowa Hospitals and
Clinics and VA Medical Center, Iowa City, Iowa

VICTORIA P. WERTH, MD
Professor of Dermatology and Medicine,
Corporal Michael J. Crescenz VA Medical
Center; Department of Dermatology,
Perelman Center for Advanced Medicine,
University of Pennsylvania School of
Medicine, Philadelphia, Pennsylvania

CHRISTOPHER M. WOLFE, DO
Division of Dermatology, Florida State
University College of Medicine, Tallahassee,
Florida

STEPHEN E. WOLVERTON, MD
Theodore Arlook Professor of Clinical
Dermatology, Department of Dermatology,
Indiana University, Indianapolis, Indiana

Contents

> The present article addresses several high-impact practice gaps affecting psoriatic patients, current practices, the barriers that prevent the delivery of optimal care, and recommendations to improve patient outcomes. Discussions of treatment, cardiovascular risk factor screening, psoriatic arthritis screening, and biologics are included. Finally, an overview of current resident exposure to psoriatic care and recommendations for improvements in resident education are made.

> Patients with skin-predominant lupus erythematosus, dermatomyositis, and morphea should be evaluated, treated, and followed by dermatologists who can take primary responsibility for their care. Many academic centers have specialized centers with dermatologists who care for these patients. Patients with skin-predominant lupus erythematosus should be followed regularly with laboratory tests to detect significant systemic disease. Antibody tests can help determine the risks for individual patients. Patients with morphea rarely progress to systemic disease, but therapies can be helpful in treating and preventing progression of disease.

> Treatment of autoimmune patients can be challenging and rewarding. These patients often remain undiagnosed for prolonged periods of time or underdiagnosed without immunologic confirmation, resulting in significant morbidity. The most important principle in management of autoimmune bullous disease is to halt blistering activity while minimizing side effects of medications, especially those caused by corticosteroids. Judicious use of systemic steroids and steroid-sparing agents are essential tools in the management of these patients. Rituximab and intravenous immunoglobulin are playing increasingly important and earlier roles in management. Understanding of and surveillance for drug side effects are critical in long-term management.

> There are several practice gaps in the evaluation and management of itch. These gaps include a dearth of objective measures of itch, infrequent use of validated patient-reported outcomes for itch, non–evidence-based treatment, and lack of consensus about the ideal workup for generalized itch. The present article reviews these gaps and presents potential solutions.

highlight common educational and practice gaps in these areas. Finally, possible solutions to these gaps are addressed.

Julie V. Schaffer

In the past 2 decades, there has been enormous progress in determining the molecular bases of genodermatoses. This progress has expanded the interface between dermatology and genetics. Integration of clinical and molecular data has simplified disease classification and highlighted relationships among conditions. However, the recent explosion in genetic knowledge has not yet been fully incorporated into clinical dermatology practice or dermatology resident education. This article highlights strategies to overcome barriers and correct practice and educational gaps, enhancing the ability of dermatologists to diagnose, counsel, evaluate, and treat patients and families affected by genodermatoses.

Stephen E. Wolverton

The term "drug reactions" is relevant to dermatology in three categories of reactions: cutaneous drug reactions without systemic features, cutaneous drug reactions with systemic features, and systemic drugs prescribed by the dermatologist with systematic adverse effects. This article uses examples from each of these categories to illustrate several important principles central to drug reaction diagnosis and management. The information presented will help clinicians attain the highest possible level of certainty before making clinical decisions.

Armand B. Cognetta Jr, Christopher M. Wolfe, David J. Goldberg, and Hyokyoung Grace Hong

Guidelines for appropriate use of superficial radiation therapy are based on decades of research; although no formal appropriate use criteria have been developed, they are warranted. Superficial radiation in the outpatient dermatologic setting is the least expensive form of radiation treatment. Although higher cure rates may be possible with Mohs surgery, this should never argue against dermatologists retaining and refining a modality, nor should we limit its use by our successors. Most important, our elderly and infirm patients should continue to benefit from superficial radiation therapy in outpatient dermatologic settings.

Murad Alam, Abigail Waldman, and Ian A. Maher

Surgery for skin cancer is a major part of clinical dermatology, and the largest single component of dermatologic surgery practice. In general, residency training in dermatology provides comprehensive training in the theory and practice of skin cancer surgery. Practicing dermatologists are similarly expert in this area, and frequently assist other medical and surgical services by managing and coordinating the care of patients with skin cancer. However, there are minor gaps in training and practice that bear scrutiny and are amenable to rectification. This article defines the current practice in surgical treatment of skin cancers by dermatologists, gaps in practice, and mechanisms to improve current surgical practice.

DERMATOLOGIC CLINICS

THE CLINICS ARE AVAILABLE ONLINE!
Access your subscription at:
www.theclinics.com

Preface
Practice Gaps and Training Gaps: Delineating What We Need to Fix

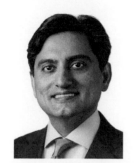

Murad Alam, MD, MSCI, MBA
Editor

The growth in medical knowledge continues unabated. This has resulted in information overload, which can overwhelm the ability of practicing clinicians to incorporate new knowledge into their day-to-day practice. This can happen not just for theoretic knowledge that is nice to know but even for pragmatic guidance that would potentially directly impact patient care.

In short, "gaps" can occur such that what is known is not communicated to frontline practitioners. The fruits of improved understanding therefore do not benefit patients. Other, similar types of gaps are also possible. For instance, researchers may fail to broach questions or problems that are of great relevance to clinicians. Here, the problem is not a lack of transmission of knowledge but a dearth of knowledge itself. Gaps can also emerge during dermatology residency, when useful information is not imparted to trainees.

Gaps occur because of obstacles, and they can be rectified by taking particular steps. The first step is to identify gaps. Next, the relevant causative obstacles and ideal corrective can be considered.

In this issue, we have invited content experts in specific areas of dermatology to think deeply about gaps in their subfields. We have asked them to identify practice gaps and training gaps, describe the obstacles that allow these to emerge, and suggest remedies that may help bridge these gaps.

Our expert contributors are free to cite the relevant literature, but the heart of each piece is their personal understanding of the limits of their content area based on years of experience. We have asked them to be brief, with a focus on the most important gaps, so that these most salient issues are easy to find and understand.

It is our hope that the creativity and incisive analysis of our contributors will stimulate work to fix these gaps.

Murad Alam, MD, MSCI, MBA
Department of Dermatology
Section of Cutaneous and Aesthetic Surgery
Northwestern University
Feinberg School of Medicine
676 North St. Clair Street
Suite 1600
Chicago, IL 60611, USA

E-mail address:
m-alam@northwestern.edu

Dermatol Clin 34 (2016) xiii
http://dx.doi.org/10.1016/j.det.2016.04.001
0733-8635/16/$ – see front matter © 2016 Published by Elsevier Inc.

Psoriasis Trends and Practice Gaps

Alice B. Gottlieb, MD, PhD*, Jacqueline E. Greb, BA, Ari M. Goldminz, MD

KEYWORDS

• Psoriasis • Psoriatic arthritis • Practice gaps • Treatment trends • Biologics • Resident education

KEY POINTS

- Psoriatic patients remain undertreated despite an increasing number of available systemic therapies, including biologics, with growing long-term safety data.
- Despite the established increased risk of cardiovascular disease risk factors and adverse outcomes among patients with psoriasis, routine screening and counseling is not a widespread practice.
- Although the importance of early psoriatic arthritis diagnosis is known, rates of detection remain less than the predicted incidence rates.
- Economic disincentives lead to limited adherence to standard of care in the treatment of psoriasis and psoriatic arthritis.
- Collaborative efforts can address the key deficiencies in psoriasis treatment, screening, and education.

INTRODUCTION

Psoriasis is a chronic, immune-mediated disorder that affects 2% to 3% of the global population. The most prevalent psoriatic disease phenotype is plaque-type, although other, less common subtypes include inverse, guttate, pustular, and erythrodermic. In addition to its cutaneous manifestations, psoriasis negatively impacts quality of life; is associated with rheumatologic, ophthalmologic, cardiac, and psychiatric comorbidities, and leads to economic burdens both for individual patients and society. The present article addresses several high-impact and clinically important practice gaps affecting the care of psoriatic patients. For each topic the authors review current

practices, the gaps and barriers that prevent the delivery of optimal care, and recommendations to improve patient outcomes.

TREATMENT
Standards of Care

Selection of an appropriate treatment regimen is tailored to individual patients based on disease severity, measured by body surface area, disease location, presence of psoriatic arthritis, impact on quality of life, and previous responses or contraindications to psoriatic therapies. Specific psoriasis treatment algorithms have been developed by leaders in the field and are previously published.[1] Topical therapies are selected as a monotherapy

Conflicts of Interest: A.B. Gottlieb currently has consulting/advisory board agreements with the following: Amgen Inc; Astellas, Akros, Centocor (Janssen), Inc; Celgene Corp; Bristol Myers Squibb Co; Beiersdorf, Inc; Abbott Labs (Abbvie); TEVA; Actelion; UCB; Novo Nordisk; Novartis; Dermipsor Ltd; Incyte; Pfizer; Canfite; Lilly; Coronado; Vertex; Karyopharm; CSL Behring Biotherapies for Life; Glaxo Smith Kline; Xenoport; Catabasis; Meiji Seika Pharma Co, Ltd; Takeda; and Mitsubishi Tanabe Pharma Development America, Inc. She has research/educational grants (paid to Tufts Medical Center) with the following: Centocor (Janssen), Amgen, Abbott (Abbvie), Novartis, Celgene, Pfizer, Lilly, Coronado, Levia, Merck, and Xenoport. J.E. Greb and A.M. Goldminz have no conflicts to report.
Department of Dermatology, Tufts Medical Center, 800 Washington Street, Box 114, Boston, MA 02111, USA
* Corresponding author.
E-mail address: Agottlieb@tuftsmedicalcenter.org

Dermatol Clin 34 (2016) 235–242
http://dx.doi.org/10.1016/j.det.2016.03.004
0733-8635/16/$ – see front matter

for localized disease but are not appropriate for more widespread cutaneous lesions, severe involvement of the palmoplantar surfaces, genitalia, scalp, or nails, and psoriatic arthritis. In these cases systemic treatments are required, such as cyclosporine, oral retinoids (in the absence of psoriatic arthritis), methotrexate, apremilast or biologic agents. Currently biologic agents are the gold standard for the systemic treatment of psoriasis and psoriatic arthritis with more rapid and complete control of disease signs and symptoms and a more favorable side effect profile.[2]

Current Practice

Despite the increasing number of highly efficacious and safe treatments for psoriasis, surveys demonstrate overall low treatment satisfaction and high noncompliance among psoriatic patients.[3,4] In a survey of 5604 patients with psoriasis or psoriatic arthritis, approximately 50% are reportedly dissatisfied with their current treatment.[5] Among patients with mild, moderate, and severe disease, one-half, one-third, and one-fifth remain untreated, respectively. Additionally, topical treatments alone were prescribed to 30% of patients with moderate disease and 21% of patients with severe disease.

Three hundred ninety-one dermatologists in North America and Europe surveyed in the Multinational Assessment of Psoriasis and Psoriatic Arthritis program demonstrated similar results.[6] Among patients with moderate to severe disease, topical monotherapy was prescribed to 54.0%, systemic therapy to 39.1%, and biologic therapy to 19.6%. Despite the US Food and Drug Administration approval of biologic agents for the treatment of psoriasis since 2003, a retrospective review of the US National Ambulatory Medical Care Survey and the National Hospital Ambulatory Medical Care Survey demonstrated no increase in the use of systemic therapy for moderate to severe psoriasis between 1993 and 2010.[7] Similarly among private practitioners in Germany, systemic treatments for psoriasis were prescribed to 31% of patients with moderate to severe psoriasis and only 58% of patients with psoriatic arthritis.[8]

Gaps

Despite a growing number of systemic agents and increasing long-term safety data for these therapies, a large number of psoriatic patients remain undertreated. Additional considerations, such as the association between psoriasis and cardiovascular (CV) disease and the cardioprotective effects of several systemic therapies, add further

importance to appropriate treatment selection. Provider- and patient-centered, clinically relevant, and adaptable outcome measures in psoriasis incorporating key domains comorbidities including CV risk and psoriatic arthritis are lacking.[9] These measures would provide more defined end points to assess treatment efficacy in clinical practice.

Barriers

In a survey conducted by dermatologists from both academic and private practice settings in Germany, self-reported confidence in prescribing systemic psoriasis treatments is low, with 76% of those polled noting that their own confidence in prescribing systemic agents limited their use.[10] Among physicians asked about the prescription of anti–tumor necrosis factor (TNF) agents, none were very confident, 9% were confident, 27% were relatively confident, 48% were uncertain, and 16% were very uncertain. Fewer than half of dermatologists reported that they were aware of the most recent guidelines 6 months after publication. Additional concerns over long-term safety, tolerability, and efficacy of systemic agents also influence prescription practices.[6]

Moreover, prescribing is influenced by the considerable time and overhead costs required for the prescription and management of systemic therapies. An example is the inefficient system of verbal and written interactions with insurance companies and pharmacies in order to obtain prior authorizations.[8] Further economic disincentives, including physician tiering, also negatively impact treatment patterns in psoriasis and other chronic conditions.[11] The cost and quality measures used to assign provider tiers fail to integrate important variables, such as disease severity, case complexity, and clearance of disease. Therefore, physicians receiving difficult referrals and treating refractory, chronic diseases that require expensive interventions are assigned worse tiers because of the higher costs of their practice. One consequence of receiving a worse tier is that patients require higher copays to see the doctor and the physician may be excluded from their tight networks. Finally, the lack of outcome measures useful in clinical practice that evaluate disease co-morbidities based on the input of both patient and provider prevents meaningful assessment of treatment effectiveness.

Recommendations for Improvement

The steps taken to address the treatment gaps in psoriasis are among the most important initiatives facing patients with psoriasis and the providers who deliver care. A group of academic and private practice German dermatologists participated in a 2-hour educational initiative focused on assisting physicians to optimize the selection of psoriasis treatments based on the most recent guidelines. Among participants, 42% reported that they would change their daily practice based on this single training session.[10] Both educational initiatives and greater incentives for the appropriate use of systemic agents are necessary. A combined educational initiative involving multiple dermatologic societies would provide the most global visibility, both for practitioners and their patients. Thoughtfully developed measures that limit disincentives for prescribing systemic therapies should be developed, for example, a code specific for the prescription of biologic agents that factors time required by ancillary staff to navigate the process from the initial prior authorization to the delivery of a medication to patients (see section Access to Biologics later). Medical practice models that integrate dermatologists, primary care physicians, physician assistants, and nurse practitioners into psoriasis management have also shown promise in improving the care that psoriatic patients receive.[12]

Finally, clinically practical, patient-centered treatment outcome measures that assess clearance of psoriasis and important psoriasis comorbidities, including CV risk and psoriatic arthritis, are needed.[9] These measures will ultimately provide meaningful feedback to providers and other stakeholders, such as payers to help achieve the standard of care in the treatment of psoriatic disease. This process is currently underway through the International Dermatology Outcome Measures (IDEOM) initiative.[13,14] The IDEOM has adapted principles defined by the Outcome Measure for Rheumatoid Arthritis Clinical Trials initiative in rheumatology that has accomplished a similar goal.[15] IDEOM outcome initiatives involve not only patients and health care providers but also regulatory agencies, pharmaceutical health economists, and payers. The two diseases currently under study are psoriasis and hidradenitis suppurativa.

CARDIOVASCULAR RISK FACTOR SCREENING
Standards

Psoriatic patients, particularly those with severe disease and those with psoriatic arthritis, have a higher prevalence of CV risk factors, including hypertension, diabetes, obesity, dyslipidemia, and insulin resistance, increasing the risk for adverse outcomes, such as coronary artery disease, myocardial infarction, stroke, and CV death.[16–20] The association between psoriasis and the proinflammatory

cascade may have a systemic effect leading to an increased risk of CV disease.[21] Treatment with anti-TNF agents and other therapies, such as methotrexate, reduce both the inflammatory burden and the risk of CV disease.[22–25] Current practice guidelines include counseling all patients with psoriasis about lifestyle modifications, smoking cessation, and monitoring for comorbidities, such as hypertension, obesity, and diabetes mellitus.[25–27] The National Psoriasis Foundation and American Heart Association also recommend screening psoriatic patients for CV risk factors beginning at 20 years of age.[28] Consensus guidelines from a European-led panel include yearly CV risk factor screening with measurements of blood pressure, body mass index, waist circumference, lipid profile, fasting glucose, glycosylated hemoglobin, and smoking status with aggressive risk factor management for patients with moderate to severe psoriasis.[29] Targets for risk factor interventions may also need to be adjusted, as psoriasis is a known independent risk factor for CV disease.[29,30] However, no such recommendations currently exist. At routine follow-up visits for psoriasis, dermatologists should provide encouragement about lifestyle modifications and regular appointments with primary care providers.[29] The positive effects of counseling by dermatologists was demonstrated in one study, showing 79.1% of psoriatic patients who were educated on their increased CV risk made subsequent lifestyle changes.[28] The dermatologist should also communicate the patients' increased CV risk to the primary care physician directly. However, when treatment of CV risk or adverse events becomes necessary, patients should seek further care and referrals from their primary care physician.

Current Practices

Psoriatic patients are screened for CV risk factors and treated for comorbid conditions, such as hypertension, less frequently than the general population.[28,31] Similarly, counseling on lifestyle modifications, such as smoking and alcohol cessation, is not a routine practice.[32] In data collected from 251 primary care physicians and cardiologists, only 45% of those surveyed were aware of the increased prevalence of CV disease risk factors and adverse outcomes among psoriatic patients.[31] In another recent study, 92% of dermatologists polled were aware of the increased risk for CV risk factors, of whom 72% were well aware of the increased risk and 20% had heard of the increased risk in limited detail.[33] However, only 13.9% of these dermatologists' patients were screened for dyslipidemia, 47.2% for obesity, 30.6% for hypertension, and 27.8% for diabetes. Additionally, just 26.9% of patients were educated about their increased CV disease risk, with the majority receiving this information from the mass media.

Gaps

Despite the established increased risk of CV risk factors and adverse CV outcomes among patients with psoriasis, both dermatologists and nondermatologists are not routinely screening for or counseling patients on CV risk factors.[32] The specific role of dermatologists and primary care physicians in the counseling and screening process of psoriatic patients is not well defined, and providers are not all aware of the CV risk associated with psoriasis.

Barriers

Among dermatologists' limitations in screening facilities and time, lack of integration of screening into the electronic medical record as well as ambivalence about the need for screening prevent the evaluation of psoriatic patients for CV risk factors.[28]

Recommendation for Improvement

The first step in increasing adherence to recommended screening for CV risk among psoriatic patients is creating an organized, collaborative approach between dermatologists, primary care physicians, cardiologists, and endocrinologists. Presentations and publications on CV risk and psoriasis should achieve a broad audience across multiple medical specialties.[34] Electronic medical records can incorporate specific screening questions and measurements for psoriatic patients to improve the adherence to practice guidelines for both counseling and routine testing. Self-assessment programs for physicians to emphasize the importance of CV risk screening among psoriatic patients would also improve screening rates.[34] Finally a systematic protocol for screening and management of CV risk factors should be established to clarify the specific role of each health care provider in the process.

SCREENING FOR PSORIATIC ARTHRITIS
Standards

Up to 40% of patients with psoriasis have an associated inflammatory, destructive arthritis, which can lead to permanent joint deformities when left untreated.[1] Psoriatic arthritis is characterized by enthesitis, dactylitis, spondylitis, and nail dystrophy and is associated with significant morbidity and impact on quality of life.[35] Among patients with psoriatic arthritis, approximately 15% initially

develop joint involvement only and 15% exhibit concurrent joint and skin findings, whereas in 70% skin manifestations are found before joint signs and symptoms. Therefore, all patients diagnosed with psoriasis should be routinely screened for arthritis.[36] Dermatologists play an important role in the diagnosis of psoriatic arthritis as cutaneous involvement typically presents before joint manifestations.

Early diagnosis and treatment of psoriatic arthritis improves clinical outcomes, limits pain, and prevents irreversible joint disease through suppression of pathogenic inflammatory signaling.[35,37–39] Patients with psoriasis should be questioned about symptoms, such as prolonged morning stiffness, joint swelling, erythema, or pain. The physical examination includes an investigation for signs of active synovitis and other associated findings, such as nail pitting.[40]

Patients should be screened for arthritis at the time of psoriasis diagnosis and at least annually thereafter.[29] Multiple psoriatic arthritis screening algorithms have been proposed, although the Classification of Psoriatic Arthritis (CASPAR) is the most widely used. CASPAR has a specificity of 99.1% and sensitivity of 87.0% and was developed as a tool for clinical research studies.[39,41] The Psoriasis Epidemiology Screening Tool was validated in the adult psoriatic population with a sensitivity of 94% and specificity of 78%.[42] Additional screening tools include Psoriatic Arthritis Screening and Evaluation with 82% sensitivity and 73% specificity and Toronto Psoriatic Arthritis Screening Questionnaire with 86.8% sensitivity and 93.1% specificity.[43,44]

Current Practices

Psoriatic arthritis is underdiagnosed because of limited frequency of screening, improper use of screening tools, and limitations in the currently available screening tools particularly in the general clinic setting.[41,45–48] It is also possible that economic disincentives decrease detection, as diagnosis of psoriatic arthritis increases overhead and puts the physician at increased risk for an unfavorable tier rating and elimination from tight networks.

Gaps

Although the importance of early diagnosis of psoriatic arthritis is known, rates of detection remain well less than the predicted incidence rates. Up to one-third of psoriatic arthritis cases are undiagnosed leading to significant increases in morbidity and decreases in health-related quality of life.[46–48]

Barriers

The absence of a time-efficient, validated, sensitive, and specific screening tool for psoriatic arthritis limits the frequency of early diagnosis and treatment.[35] Additional barriers include limited patient awareness of the significance and prevalence of psoriatic arthritis, lack of confidence among dermatologists in evaluating and detecting joint disease, the broad range of psoriatic arthritis manifestations, and the overlap between psoriatic arthritis and other rheumatologic conditions.[6]

Recommendations for Improvement

The creation of a time-effective, validated screening tool with high sensitivity and specificity for the detection of psoriatic arthritis is needed to improve the care provided to the psoriatic population. Educational initiatives emphasizing to patients the importance of annual screening, early diagnosis, and intervention as well as workshops to instruct dermatologists on recommended screening practices and techniques are needed. Routine questions on psoriatic arthritis that appear in the electronic medical record for all psoriatic patients would also promote screening.[40] Limiting economic disincentives for the diagnosis and treatment of psoriatic arthritis may also improve detection and treatment patterns. Finally, an interdisciplinary approach, for example, with combined rheumatology-dermatology clinics, would lead to higher detection rates of psoriatic arthritis.

ACCESS TO BIOLOGICS
Standards

After the introduction of biologic therapies for the treatment of psoriasis, patients have been provided more effective therapies with improved safety profiles compared with the traditional systemic agents, such as methotrexate or cyclosporine. Use of these biologic agents is associated with increased patient-reported treatment satisfaction and superior patient- and physician-measured outcomes. Six biologics are US Food and Drug Administration approved for treatment of psoriasis, including etanercept, adalimumab, infliximab, alefacept, secukinumab and ixekizumab. Golimumab and certolizumab are approved for psoriatic arthritis, whereas ustekinumab is approved for both psoriasis and psoriatic arthritis. Eligibility for biologics in the United States is based on the clinical severity of psoriatic disease or the associated impact on quality of life.[49] Predominantly, clinical research parameters include moderate to severe disease, such as a measured Psoriasis Area and Severity Index greater than 10 or body surface area greater than 10%,

physician global assessment, presence of psoriatic arthritis, or impact on daily life including a measured Dermatology Life Quality Index greater than 10. Skin involvement of high-impact areas, including the head, neck, palms, soles, or genitalia, is also considered. In addition, patients typically require a contraindication or previous failure of a traditional systemic treatment, such as methotrexate, because of the current high cost of biologics.

Current Practices

Although the use of biologics has increased since their introduction, they remain underutilized even in appropriate clinical contexts. The Multinational Assessment of Psoriasis and Psoriatic Arthritis survey, which randomly sampled dermatologists from Canada, the United States, France, Germany, Italy, Spain, and the United Kingdom, demonstrated that 19.6% of patients with psoriasis with moderate to severe psoriasis and 30.6% of patients with psoriatic arthritis were prescribed biologics.[6] Despite the higher cost of biologic therapies compared with traditional systemic agents, improved disease control achieved with biologics limits health care expenditures,[50] which includes fewer outpatient visits and inpatient hospitalizations for psoriatic patients.

Gaps

Biologics continue to be underutilized despite their favorable efficacy and safety data. Issues surrounding cost, insurance coverage, physician reimbursement, and access limit their use.

Barriers

In a questionnaire of psoriatic patients on biologic therapy, the most commonly cited obstacles to biologic access included negotiations with insurance companies and the ability to fill their prescription with the pharmacy.[51] Other factors associated with difficulty in obtaining biologics included younger age (<55 years old), lower income (<$100,000/y), and lack of health insurance. The annual out-of-pocket expenditure for biologics was $557 with a range of $0 to 7000 and median of $180. Economics indeed are among the key barriers to the use of biologics.[52] Among physicians surveyed in the United Kingdom, 40% cited funding as a major obstacle in their ability to prescribe biologics.[53] Additionally, hospitals and clinics are not always fully reimbursed for the cost of biologics; their physicians and staff are not compensated for the time involved with prescribing these medications.[52] In these surveys, patient- and physician-reported safety concerns were consistently less significant than economic ones. Again, physicians using biologics are at increased risk for being assigned unfavorable tiers and for being excluded from tight networks.

Recommendation for Improvement

The central issues that should be addressed to improve prescription practices of biologics include physician education (see Treatment section earlier), reductions in the costs associated with biologic agents, limiting economic disincentives, and streamlining of the steps required to prescribe these medications. Many dermatologists have not received formal training in the use of biologics, and a coordinated effort focusing on resident education would be beneficial (see Education section). As additional, more effective biologics and competing bio-similar agents are introduced, the cost of first-generation biologics may be reduced. Finally, prescription of biologics requires both the training of support staff and a significant investment of their time. Involvement of multiple entities, including academic centers and pharmaceutical companies, in the form of central processing offices can provide additional support to patients and prescribers. Additional measures to improve the process may include a prescribing and authorization service that interfaces directly with the electronic medical record as well as more consistent guidelines imposed on payers for what is required for approval of biologics. Advocacy by interested patient and health care provider organizations needs to be increased in order to educate payers on the severity of psoriasis and its comorbidities and the need for adequate treatment. These organizations should lobby payers to include case mix and clinical outcomes and not just predominantly costs when tiering physicians or choosing physicians for their networks.

RESIDENT EDUCATION
Standards

Clinical experience in a high-volume psoriasis clinic that includes management of complex patients under the supervision of a psoriasis specialist provides residents with a range of abilities in the evaluation, counseling, management, and monitoring of psoriatic patients. In this setting they will become familiar with rapidly updated guidelines, new trends in the field, and how to assess patients for psoriatic arthritis and other comorbidities. In particular, it is important that residents gain comfort with biologics, as utilization is correlated with experience in training and these agents have the unique ability to clear patients with resistant moderate to severe disease. Therefore, it is essential that residents are involved in all aspects of prescribing biologics and monitoring

patients while they are treated. If possible, residents should also be exposed to infliximab infusion clinics, although these are few in number in the United States.

Current Education

Among US-trained residents, there is variable exposure to the use of biologics and specialized psoriasis clinics that manage complex patients. Comfort with counseling psoriatic patients, an important aspect of their care, is also limited among residents. A recent questionnaire surveyed 92 US dermatology residents about their knowledge of screening and counseling psoriatic patients. Among these residents, 76%, 80%, and 94% of participants were aware of the impact of alcohol, tobacco, and obesity, respectively, on psoriasis, whereas 48%, 55%, and 63% of participants indicated they were confident or very confident counseling about behavioral changes for alcohol, tobacco, and obesity, respectively.[32] Residents were uncertain whether the patients' dermatologist or primary care physician was responsible for screening and counseling on these behaviors.

Gaps

As psoriatic patients will ultimately be a significant proportion of residents' practices, gaps in exposure are important to address. The level of comfort prescribing systemic agents and counseling patients in independent practice is directly correlated with experience during residency. Bridging this core educational gap through a multifaceted approach is essential to optimize care delivered to patients.

Barriers

Access to specialized psoriasis clinics and outpatient infusion centers represents a significant barrier in residency training in psoriasis. Lack of this exposure limits prescribing practices and compounds the current deficiencies in the use of systemic agents in psoriasis and the appropriate counseling of patients about comorbidities, such as CV disease.

Recommendations for Improvement

To improve access to specialized psoriasis clinics and facilitate instruction by leaders in the field, opportunities to participate in electives and other learning sessions should be well publicized. Through short 1- to 2-week clinical rotations at preapproved sites, residents will gain a robust exposure to all aspects of psoriatic care. Other resources could include live or taped lecture series with leaders in the field. Resident participation in the processes required to prescribe biologic agents, such as prior authorizations, should be encouraged. Finally instruction in counseling and motivational interviewing for behavior change instruction would provide the dermatologists of the future with additional tools to enhance their interactions with their psoriatic patients.

REFERENCES

1. Gottlieb A, Korman NJ, Gordon KB, et al. Guidelines of care for the management of psoriasis and psoriatic arthritis: section 2. Psoriatic arthritis: overview and guidelines of care for treatment with an emphasis on the biologics. J Am Acad Dermatol 2008;58(5):851–64.

2. Rustin MH. Long-term safety of biologics in the treatment of moderate-to-severe plaque psoriasis: review of current data. Br J Dermatol 2012; 167(Suppl 3):3–11.

3. Stern RS, Nijsten T, Feldman SR, et al. Psoriasis is common, carries a substantial burden even when not extensive, and is associated with widespread treatment dissatisfaction. J Investig Dermatol Symp Proc 2004;9(2):136–9.

4. Richards HL, Fortune DG, O'Sullivan TM, et al. Patients with psoriasis and their compliance with medication. J Am Acad Dermatol 1999;41(4):581–3.

5. Armstrong AW, Robertson AD, Wu J, et al. Undertreatment, treatment trends, and treatment dissatisfaction among patients with psoriasis and psoriatic arthritis in the United States: findings from the National Psoriasis Foundation surveys, 2003-2011. JAMA Dermatol 2013;149(10):1180–5.

6. van de Kerkhof PC, Reich K, Kavanaugh A, et al. Physician perspectives in the management of psoriasis and psoriatic arthritis: results from the population-based Multinational Assessment of Psoriasis and Psoriatic Arthritis survey. J Eur Acad Dermatol Venereol 2015;29(10):2002–10.

7. Shaw MK, Davis SA, Feldman SR, et al. Trends in systemic psoriasis treatment therapies from 1993 through 2010. J Drugs Dermatol 2014;13(8):917–20.

8. Nast A, Reytan N, Rosumeck S, et al. Low prescription rate for systemic treatments in the management of severe psoriasis vulgaris and psoriatic arthritis in dermatological practices in Berlin and Brandenburg, Germany: results from a patient registry. J Eur Acad Dermatol Venereol 2008;22(11):1337–42.

9. Kim N, Gottlieb AB. Outcome measures in psoriasis and psoriatic arthritis. Curr Dermatol Rep 2013; 2:159–63.

10. Nast A, Erdmann R, Pathirana D, et al. Translating psoriasis treatment guidelines into clinical practice - the need for educational interventions and strategies for broad dissemination. J Eval Clin Pract 2008;14(5): 803–6.

11. Freedman JD, Gottlieb AB, Lizzul PF. Physician performance measurement: tiered networks and dermatology (an opportunity and a challenge). J Am Acad Dermatol 2011;64(6):1164–9.

12. Palmer D, El Miedany Y. Biological nurse specialist: goodwill to good practice. Br J Nurs 2010;19(8): 477–80.

13. Gottlieb AB, Levin AA, Armstrong AW, et al. The International Dermatology Outcome Measures Group: formation of patient-centered outcome measures in dermatology. J Am Acad Dermatol 2015;72(2):345–8.

14. Gottlieb AB, Levin AA. The International Dermatology Outcome Measures Group: update from the GRAPPA 2014 annual meeting. J Rheumatol 2015; 42(6):1027–8.

15. Tugwell P, Boers M, Brooks P, et al. OMERACT: an international initiative to improve outcome measurement in rheumatology. Trials 2007;8:38.

16. Jamnitski A, Symmons D, Peters MJ, et al. Cardiovascular comorbidities in patients with psoriatic arthritis: a systematic review. Ann Rheum Dis 2013; 72(2):211–6.

17. Gottlieb AB, Dann F. Comorbidities in patients with psoriasis. Am J Med 2009;122(12):1150.e1–9.

18. Neimann AL, Shin DB, Wang X, et al. Prevalence of cardiovascular risk factors in patients with psoriasis. J Am Acad Dermatol 2006;55(5):829–35.

19. Gelfand JM, Troxel AB, Lewis JD, et al. The risk of mortality in patients with psoriasis: results from a population-based study. Arch Dermatol 2007; 143(12):1493–9.

20. Boehncke S, Thaci D, Beschmann H, et al. Psoriasis patients show signs of insulin resistance. Br J Dermatol 2007;157(6):1249–51.

21. Hamminga EA, van der Lely AJ, Neumann HA, et al. Chronic inflammation in psoriasis and obesity: implications for therapy. Med Hypotheses 2006;67(4): 768–73.

22. Prodanovich S, Kirsner RS, Kravetz JD, et al. Association of psoriasis with coronary artery, cerebrovascular, and peripheral vascular diseases and mortality. Arch Dermatol 2009;145(6):700–3.

23. Sommer DM, Jenisch S, Suchan M, et al. Increased prevalence of the metabolic syndrome in patients with moderate to severe psoriasis. Arch Dermatol Res 2006;298(7):321–8.

24. Boehncke S, Salgo R, Garbaraviciene J, et al. Effective continuous systemic therapy of severe plaque-type psoriasis is accompanied by amelioration of biomarkers of cardiovascular risk: results of a prospective longitudinal observational study. J Eur Acad Dermatol Venereol 2011;25(10):1187–93.

25. Famenini S, Sako EY, Wu JJ. Effect of treating psoriasis on cardiovascular co-morbidities: focus on TNF inhibitors. Am J Clin Dermatol 2014;15(1):45–50.

26. Friedewald VE, Cather JC, Gelfand JM, et al. AJC editor's consensus: psoriasis and coronary artery disease. Am J Cardiol 2008;102(12):1631–43.

27. Armstrong AW, Harskamp CT, Armstrong EJ. The association between psoriasis and obesity: a systematic review and meta-analysis of observational studies. Nutr Diabetes 2012;2:e54.

28. Kimball AB, Gladman D, Gelfand JM, et al. National Psoriasis Foundation clinical consensus on psoriasis comorbidities and recommendations for screening. J Am Acad Dermatol 2008;58(6):1031–42.

29. Strohal R, Kirby B, Puig L, et al. Psoriasis beyond the skin: an expert group consensus on the management of psoriatic arthritis and common co-morbidities in patients with moderate-to-severe psoriasis. J Eur Acad Dermatol Venereol 2014;28(12):1661–9.

30. Peters MJ, Symmons DP, McCarey D, et al. EULAR evidence-based recommendations for cardiovascular risk management in patients with rheumatoid arthritis and other forms of inflammatory arthritis. Ann Rheum Dis 2010;69(2):325–31.

31. Parsi KK, Brezinski EA, Lin TC, et al. Are patients with psoriasis being screened for cardiovascular risk factors? A study of screening practices and awareness among primary care physicians and cardiologists. J Am Acad Dermatol 2012;67(3):357–62.

32. Adler BL, Krausz AE, Tian J, et al. Modifiable lifestyle factors in psoriasis: screening and counseling practices among dermatologists and dermatology residents in academic institutions. J Am Acad Dermatol 2014;71(5):1028–9.

33. Lee MK, Kim HS, Cho EB, et al. A study of awareness and screening behavior of cardiovascular risk factors in patients with psoriasis and dermatologists. Ann Dermatol 2015;27(1):59–65.

34. Gist DL, Bhushan R, Hamarstrom E, et al. Impact of a performance improvement CME activity on the care and treatment of patients with psoriasis. J Am Acad Dermatol 2015;72(3):516–23.

35. Lloyd P, Ryan C, Menter A. Psoriatic arthritis: an update. Arthritis 2012;2012:176298.

36. Gladman DD, Shuckett R, Russell ML, et al. Psoriatic arthritis (PSA)–an analysis of 220 patients. Q J Med 1987;62(238):127–41.

37. Theander E, Husmark T, Alenius GM, et al. Early psoriatic arthritis: short symptom duration, male gender and preserved physical functioning at presentation predict favourable outcome at 5-year follow-up. Results from the Swedish Early Psoriatic Arthritis Register (SwePsA). Ann Rheum Dis 2014; 73(2):407–13.

38. Kirkham B, de Vlam K, Li W, et al. Early treatment of psoriatic arthritis is associated with improved patient-reported outcomes: findings from the etanercept PRESTA trial. Clin Exp Rheumatol 2015;33(1):11–9.

39. Coates LC, Navarro-Coy N, Brown SR, et al. The TICOPA protocol (TIght COntrol of Psoriatic Arthritis): a randomised controlled trial to compare intensive management versus standard care in early psoriatic arthritis. BMC Musculoskelet Disord 2013; 14:101.

40. Mease PJ, Armstrong AW. Managing patients with psoriatic disease: the diagnosis and pharmacologic treatment of psoriatic arthritis in patients with psoriasis. Drugs 2014;74(4):423–41.

41. Taylor W, Gladman D, Helliwell P, et al. Classification criteria for psoriatic arthritis: development of new criteria from a large international study. Arthritis Rheum 2006;54(8):2665–73.

42. The assessment and management of psoriasis. 2012. Available at: guidance.nice.org.uk/cg153. Accessed July 14, 2015.

43. Husni ME, Meyer KH, Cohen DS, et al. The PASE questionnaire: pilot-testing a psoriatic arthritis screening and evaluation tool. J Am Acad Dermatol 2007;57(4):581–7.

44. Gladman DD, Schentag CT, Tom BD, et al. Development and initial validation of a screening questionnaire for psoriatic arthritis: the Toronto Psoriatic Arthritis Screen (ToPAS). Ann Rheum Dis 2009;68(4):497–501.

45. Ganatra B, Manoharan D, Akhras V. Use of a validated screening tool for psoriatic arthritis in dermatology clinics. BMJ Qual Improv Rep 2015;4(1).

46. Gladman DD, Antoni C, Mease P, et al. Psoriatic arthritis: epidemiology, clinical features, course, and outcome. Ann Rheum Dis 2005;64(Suppl 2):ii14–7.

47. Haroon M, Kirby B, FitzGerald O. High prevalence of psoriatic arthritis in patients with severe psoriasis with suboptimal performance of screening questionnaires. Ann Rheum Dis 2013;72(5):736–40.

48. Mease PJ, Gladman DD, Papp KA, et al. Prevalence of rheumatologist-diagnosed psoriatic arthritis in patients with psoriasis in European/North American dermatology clinics. J Am Acad Dermatol 2013; 69(5):729–35.

49. Smith CH, Anstey AV, Barker JN, et al. British Association of Dermatologists' guidelines for biologic interventions for psoriasis 2009. Br J Dermatol 2009; 161(5):987–1019.

50. Bhosle MJ, Feldman SR, Camacho FT, et al. Medication adherence and health care costs associated with biologics in Medicaid-enrolled patients with psoriasis. J Dermatolog Treat 2006;17(5):294–301.

51. Kamangar F, Isip L, Bhutani T, et al. How psoriasis patients perceive, obtain, and use biologic agents: survey from an academic medical center. J Dermatolog Treat 2013;24(1):13–24.

52. Nast A, Mrowietz U, Kragballe K, et al. Barriers to the prescription of systemic therapies for moderate-to-severe psoriasis–a multinational cross-sectional study. Arch Dermatol Res 2013;305(10):899–907.

53. Eedy DJ, Griffiths CE, Chalmers RJ, et al. Care of patients with psoriasis: an audit of U.K. services in secondary care. Br J Dermatol 2009;160(3):557–64.

Practice and Educational Gaps in Lupus, Dermatomyositis, and Morphea

CrossMark

Nicole M. Fett, MD, MSCE[a], David Fiorentino, MD, PhD[b],
Victoria P. Werth, MD[c,d],*

KEYWORDS

- Lupus • Dermatomyositis • Morphea • Practice • Educational gaps

KEY POINTS

- Patients with skin-predominant lupus erythematosus, dermatomyositis, and morphea should be evaluated, treated, and followed by dermatologists who can take primary responsibility for their care.
- Many academic centers have specialized centers with dermatologists who care for these patients.
- Patients with skin-predominant lupus erythematosus should be followed regularly with laboratory tests, including urinalysis, to detect significant systemic disease.
- Patients with dermatomyositis should be appropriately evaluated for the presence of lung, muscle disease, and cancer. Antibody tests can help determine the risks for individual patients.
- Patients with morphea may develop joint contractures and limb length discrepancy, which may significantly affect mobility. Additionally, patients with morphea often have associated pain and itch which affect quality of life. Treatment of morphea is targeted to prevent functional and emotional limitations.

LUPUS ERYTHEMATOSUS: BEST PRACTICES
Clinical and Laboratory Assessment

Best practices in cutaneous lupus erythematosus (CLE) include recognizing the clinical presentations of specific subsets of CLE (localized and generalized discoid LE [DLE], subacute cutaneous LE, acute cutaneous LE). There should be recognition that more than one subset may be seen in a given patient, assessment of whether the disease is active, and documentation of the degree of skin disease activity. Also, recognition of the extent of cutaneous damage is important, particularly if there is ongoing activity that needs aggressive treatment because of continued risk for scarring and dyspigmentation. The impact on quality of life should be assessed. There should be recognition of the importance of considering other potential diagnoses and the frequent need for initial documentation by skin biopsy to rule out mimickers and assure the need for proper

Funding Sources: This work was supported by the United States Department of Veterans Affairs (Veterans Health Administration, Office of Research and Development and Biomedical Laboratory Research (VA ORD 5 I01 BX000706-04) and Development) and the National Institutes of Health NIH R21 AR066286 for V.P. Werth.
Disclosure: The copyright for the CLASI and CDASI is owned by the University of Pennsylvania.
[a] Department of Dermatology, Center for Health and Healing, Oregon Health & Science University, 3303 Southwest Bond Avenue, 16th Floor, Portland, OR 97239, USA; [b] Department of Dermatology, Stanford University School of Medicine, 450 Broadway, Redwood City, CA 94063, USA; [c] Corporal Michael J. Crescenz VA Medical Center, Philadelphia, PA, USA; [d] Department of Dermatology, Perelman Center for Advanced Medicine, University of Pennsylvania School of Medicine, Suite 1-330A, 3400 Civic Center Boulevard, Philadelphia, PA 19104, USA
* Corresponding author. Department of Dermatology, Perelman Center for Advanced Medicine, Suite 1-330A, 3400 Civic Center Boulevard, Philadelphia, PA 19104.
E-mail address: werth@mail.med.upenn.edu

derm.theclinics.com

long-term management. It should be recognized that subacute cutaneous lupus is frequently associated with the use of certain medications, and these should be reviewed and stopped if potentially a trigger. Patients should also be carefully assessed by history for systemic symptoms, and laboratory tests should be assessed to rule out systemic disease. These initial laboratory tests should include antinuclear antibodies (ANA), complete blood count (CBC), and urinalysis. Proteinuria, if present, should be further quantified with spot protein: creatinine ratios, and if abnormal, then 24-hour urine for protein quantification. If there is an indication of systemic features, then double-stranded DNA (dsDNA), C3, C4, anticardiolipin antibodies, and complete metabolic panel should be evaluated. Anti-Smith antibodies can be obtained if the diagnosis of lupus is unclear, because it is a specific but not sensitive antibody for diagnosing LE. If patients are contemplating pregnancy, determining the presence of anti-SSA and anti–SSB antibodies is done because pregnant patients are managed differently because of the risk of neonatal lupus if they have these antibodies. Dermatologists should evaluate patients with CLE for the presence of significant systemic disease and manage patients with skin-predominant disease. They should provide ongoing assessments for development of systemic disease, refer patients when indicated because of serious systemic findings, but assume responsibility for long-term care or refer patients to centers with dermatologists who care for such patients. Dermatologists provide optimal skin care and preventive assessment of patients with skin-predominant disease.

Patient Education and Treatment

Patients should receive counseling about broad-spectrum sunscreen use, sun avoidance, and use of sun-protective clothing. Smoking cessation should be strongly recommended, and patients should be given suggestions on how best to pursue this. If disease is mild, topical therapy should be instituted. If there is evidence that skin disease is severe or progressive, systemic treatment should be recommended with antimalarials, immunosuppressives, thalidomide, and lenalidomide. Patients with depression or anxiety may need referral to psychiatry.

Longitudinal Care

Disease activity and damage should be monitored with photographs and skin disease severity scores, such as the Cutaneous Lupus Erythematosus Disease Area and Severity Index (CLASI), to assess disease progression.[1] Patients should be counseled that CLE can progress to systemic disease. They need monitoring based on the type of CLE, evidence of systemic lupus erythematosus (SLE), and length of stable CLE.[2] Many patients meet SLE criteria but have predominantly skin findings. These patients need to be reassured that their disease is mild, but they need to be monitored to make sure their disease does not progress to organ-threatening disease. This monitoring should be done by dermatologists, and includes CBC, urinalysis, and, when indicated, dsDNA and complement levels. This testing should be done at least yearly, even for patients with localized DLE, because they can progress to organ-threatening SLE including glomerulonephritis at any point. Patients with SLE tendencies should be monitored more frequently. Eye examinations should be done yearly, at the most, if patients are on hydroxychloroquine.[3] Patients on chloroquine should be monitored every 4 to 6 months. Patients with evidence of systemic disease may require ongoing care with antimalarials to prevent disease progression.[4]

Cutaneous Lupus Erythematosus: Estimate of Current Practice

There is no systematic collection of data related to current practice; but many patients are referred to dermatologists at academic centers, frequently by rheumatologists who have been initially referred to the patients from dermatologists for their skin-predominant disease. This referral to rheumatologists is not necessary or in the best interest of patients in terms of managing their CLE. Routine monitoring of laboratory test results is not always done when patients are followed by dermatologists for localized disease. Frequently there is no organized method for monitoring disease progression/improvement, and patients do not get systemic therapy when indicated for their CLE.

Lupus Erythematosus: Gaps

CLE does not automatically progress to SLE, but patients need baseline and ongoing monitoring. In addition, objective skin disease monitoring and evaluation of quality of life is needed. Dermatologists can do this, but frequently these patients are referred to rheumatologists when a diagnosis of CLE is made before any further evaluation or systemic treatment. The practice gaps related to lack of complete workup for systemic disease and systemic treatment of skin disease includes knowledge and skill gaps that are addressable. There are also attitude gaps, such as a dermatologist's hesitancy to screen for systemic disease and/or objectively assess and manage LE skin disease with systemic agents. As discussed, many dermatologists reflexively refer these patients to a rheumatologist, which is also an attitude gap.

Although recommendations for how to monitor patients with SLE exist, recommendations for monitoring patients with CLE or skin-predominant disease are less clear and must be individualized at the current time based on the severity of disease and systemic findings, with recognition that routine laboratory test results monitoring is required for patients with skin-predominant disease.[2,5] Treatment recommendations for CLE are eminence based rather than Delphi-derived recommendations.[2,6–8] However, increasingly controlled trials or observational studies using the CLASI are now providing evidence for approaches to treatment that can begin to address information and knowledge gaps.[9–12] Much work is needed to improve the evidence for current approaches to evaluation and treatment as well as to develop consensus guidelines that determine best practices for CLE.

The barriers related to attitude gaps are best addressed by changes in education of residents and practitioners by increasing interaction with rheumatology, a cultural/attitude change in dermatology related to providing ongoing care for sick patients with skin-predominant CLE, and an awareness of the presence of specialized dermatologists in centers that frequently care for such patients where such patients can be referred.

Dermatomyositis: Best Practices

Clinical and laboratory assessment

A vision of best practices in the management of dermatomyositis (DM) entails both improving specific knowledge and skills of the average practicing dermatologist as well as the development of evidence-based guidelines that will help guide even the most seasoned experts. At a minimum, dermatologists should play the major role in recognition, assessment, interpretation, and management of the cutaneous signs of the disease. Dermatologists should consider the diagnosis in cases not only with classic cutaneous findings but also in those with more atypical presentations that mimic hand dermatitis, psoriasis, or lupus. Dermoscopy should be used regularly to detect periungual telangiectasias, a sensitive marker for DM. It should be common knowledge for a dermatologist that a significant proportion of patients with DM will never develop detectable muscle inflammation. Our specialty needs to also appreciate the spectrum of histologic changes in DM skin biopsies and not rule out the diagnosis if

interface dermatitis is not reported[13] while at the same time advocating for the importance of biopsies for ruling out mimickers of DM. The dermatologist should understand how to use serologic testing to diagnose DM and order these tests on all patients with any skin eruption that could be consistent with DM; this includes not depending on a positive ANA for diagnosis as well as routinely ordering the recently described DM-specific auto-antibodies.[14] All dermatologists should be able to identify typical signs and symptoms associated with active (vs damaged) skin disease in order to optimize therapy and prevent unnecessary use of immunosuppressants.

Screening for systemic disease

In a best practice scenario, dermatologists would always appropriately screen their patients with DM for internal malignancy. This screening includes an understanding of the time (within 1–2 years of first DM symptom) and patient population (clinical and laboratory risk factors) that are most appropriate to conduct such a search. Dermatologists should understand how advanced age, male sex, cutaneous necrosis, and autoantibodies inform risk for internal malignancy.[15] Dermatologists should be prepared to use not only the history, physical examination, and age-appropriate cancer screening but also more aggressive testing (such as computed tomography or traditional cancer screening tests out of the appropriate age window) in order to identify the patients with internal malignancy.

In addition, all dermatologists should at least be able to effectively screen patients for evidence of extracutaneous (systemic) disease in DM. Myositis should be assessed by evaluating not only for weakness but also asking about myalgia, dysphagia, and dysphonia as well as performing basic muscle strength testing in the clinic. All patients should be regularly screened with muscle enzymes (creatine kinase, aldolase, lactate dehydrogenase, aspartate transaminase, alanine transaminase) every 3 to 6 months; however, every physician should recognize that significant muscle inflammation can occur even if these tests are normal and should understand that electromyography and/or MRI should be performed in this setting in patients with clinically significant weakness or dysphagia. Dermatologists should regularly (perhaps annually) screen their patients for interstitial lung disease by ordering and interpreting annual pulmonary function testing. They should be able to identify clinical (mechanics hands, Raynaud, cutaneous ulcerations) and laboratory (antisynthetase or anti-melanoma differentiation-associated protein 5 (MDA5) autoantibodies) risk factors for interstitial lung disease and, in high-risk patients, consider more frequent or aggressive screening.

Patient counseling and treatment

Optimal patient management by a dermatologist would include both counseling and effective therapy for their skin disease. Patients should be counseled regarding the risk of internal malignancy, extracutaneous disease (especially muscle and lung involvement), and specific skin complications, such as ulceration and calcinosis. Ideally each provider would use a simple DM-specific skin activity instrument (such as the Cutaneous Dermatomyositis Activity and Severity Index) with his or her patients in order to quantify skin disease activity and rationally evaluate the treatment regimen.[16] Every dermatologist should assess how DM skin disease is impacting patients' quality of life in order to avoid the pitfall of undertreating skin disease and should appreciate that the topical therapies alone will not be sufficient skin therapy for most patients. Thus, they would be comfortable prescribing and safely monitoring traditional and biological systemic agents (including antimalarials, methotrexate, mycophenolate mofetil, leflunomide, and intravenous immunoglobulin) or be willing and able to refer patients to local *dermatologists* that can do so. *Dermatologists should take the role as primary provider for those patients with DM with skin-predominant disease* but understand when referral to other subspecialties (eg, rheumatology, pulmonology, neurology) is warranted if patients have evidence of clinically significant extracutaneous disease.

Dermatomyositis: Estimate Current Practice

No data exist to reflect the current practice of how dermatologists manage patients with DM. Based on the authors' experience, many dermatologists do not consider the diagnosis of DM in cases that either do not present with classic clinical (such as Gottron papules) or histologic (interface dermatitis) changes; thus, patients without obvious muscle weakness may not be diagnosed in a timely manner. These patients are also missed because many dermatologists are not familiar with the fact that DM-specific antibodies have now been described that can characterize 80% to 90% of all patients. There is a lack of awareness of when and how patients should be evaluated for cancer as well as lung disease and myositis. Many dermatologists do not know how to interpret autoantibody testing with regard to prognosis and how that can, at a minimum, aid in the counseling of our patients. Many patients are not offered systemic therapy for their skin disease; even those with skin-predominant disease are often referred

to other specialties (especially rheumatologists) when optimal skin care and systemic screening should be performed by the medical dermatologist.

Dermatomyositis Gaps

The gaps in practice that exist in managing patients with DM fall into 2 categories: First, there are gaps that can be addressed via professional education, practice skills enhancement, and attitude. The second type of gap exists because of a paucity of data or commercially available testing to help guide even the most experienced of practitioners. For example, many dermatologists are simply not aware of the clinical and histologic heterogeneity that can be seen in DM. In addition, new information regarding novel antibodies has been published at a rapid rate over the past several years. These gaps are quantitative knowledge gaps that are addressable and more accurately represent communication gaps. There are also attitude gaps, such as a dermatologist's hesitancy to screen for systemic disease and/or manage DM skin disease with systemic agents. In addition, many dermatologists reflexively refer these patients to a rheumatologist, as discussed earlier, which is also an attitude gap. A major practice gap that needs to be closed is the underutilization of autoantibody testing in the clinical practice; this partly stems from a lack of communication to the practicing dermatologist but also results from unavailability of testing in the clinical setting (see later discussion).

There are several barriers that need to be addressed before these gaps can be closed. First, as a specialty, we need to clarify and communicate with our dermatology colleagues what a consensus vision of best practice specifically looks like. This task would be best achieved by establishing consensus among recognized international dermatology experts regarding cutaneous diagnostic criteria for DM, timing and methodology for screening for malignancy and extracutaneous disease, and a management algorithm for skin disease. Initially these conferences can provide tentative guidelines based on experience and opinion but ultimately should specifically define what research studies or data are needed to better inform future guidelines. This task would include creating and validating cutaneous diagnostic criteria for DM, identifying which malignancy screening tests should be used for which specific populations, and performing comparative efficacy assessments of systemic therapies for skin disease. One current barrier that exists is the lack of a reliable, quantitative, commercially available manner in which to test patients for autoantibody against DM-specific targets; these tests are largely described in a research setting, and the few commercially available options have unknown sensitivity and specificity. This will require a large effort, likely international, to harmonize and validate consensus methodologies for each of these antibodies and make them commercially available to the practicing clinician.

Morphea: best practices

To date, no best practices have been established for morphea. The Childhood Arthritis and Rheumatology Research Alliance (CARRA) has published a consensus treatment and assessment plan for children with morphea.[17] CARRA's hope is that all pediatric rheumatologists will treat and assess childhood morphea the same, which will allow for comparative effectiveness studies and ultimately the establishment of best practices. The Morphea Research Alliance (MRA) is striving to establish consensus treatment and assessment plans for adults with morphea.

The following practices are recommended by experts in morphea. The patient history should document time of onset, rapidity of lesion growth/new lesion onset, possible triggers (trauma, radiation), symptoms associated with the morphea lesions, the impact of the disease on quality of life, a history assessing for other comorbid autoimmune diseases, and a family history assessing for autoimmunity.

A full-body skin examination (including the oral and genital mucosa given the co-occurrence of mucosal involvement) of patients with morphea is helpful to assess the extent of involvement and to categorize patients' morphea subtype (circumscribed, generalized, linear, mixed, pansclerotic)[18] and depth of involvement (dermal, deep dermal, subcutaneous fat, muscle, bone). The subtype of morphea and depth of involvement are important factors in therapeutic decisions and prognosis counseling. The physical examination, along with history, can be used to establish whether the disease is in the active phase (ie, patients are developing new morphea lesions, having expansion of existing lesions, or have erythema or violaceous discoloration surrounding the lesions).[19] Active disease is treatable with immunosuppression. Morphea in the damage phase (stable number of plaques, no expansion of the plaques, hyperpigmented or sclerotic plaques without signs of inflammation) will not improve with immunosuppression. Physical examination should also be used to assess for range of motion in all involved joints. Any limitations should be documented for clinical monitoring and patients with range of motion limitations referred to physical therapy and/or occupational therapy. Physical examination should also be used to help rule out systemic sclerosis. (Sclerodactyly, nail fold capillary changes, and Raynaud's phenomenon are early signs of systemic sclerosis that are not present in patients with morphea.)

There are no autoantibodies that are specific to morphea; therefore, autoantibody tests are not helpful in the diagnosis or prognosis of morphea. Assessment of autoantibodies specific to systemic sclerosis (anticentromere, antitopoisomerase, anti–RNA polymerase III) is unnecessary in the evaluation of patients with morphea. The diagnosis of systemic sclerosis requires a combination of physical examination findings, Raynaud phenomenon, and autoantibodies. Positive systemic sclerosis–specific antibodies in isolation (ie, in patients without sclerodactyly, Raynaud phenomenon, and nail fold capillary changes) are not helpful diagnostically and are most likely to be false-positive results. Biopsy is not required to make a diagnosis of classic morphea; however, biopsy may be helpful in nontraditional presentations.

Objective measurements of disease activity (full-body photographs or body maps with locations and measurements or the Localized Scleroderma Assessment Tool [LoSCAT][19]) should occur at each visit to monitor response to therapy. Children with head and neck morphea should be evaluated by ophthalmology to assess for asymptomatic ocular involvement (which is treatable and may prevent vision loss).[20] Although linear morphea of the head and neck has been associated with involvement of the central nervous system, MRI findings have not been correlated with symptoms and signs of central nervous system (CNS) involvement.[21] Therefore, only children with signs or symptoms of CNS involvement should undergo MRI.

Morphea treatment decisions need to take into account the disease subtype, depth of involvement, and quality-of-life impairments. In general, patients with active deep linear morphea, active deep mixed variant morphea, active deep generalized morphea, and active pansclerotic morphea should be treated with systemic steroids (a 3-month taper) and methotrexate (ideally for a duration of 2 years) in an attempt to prevent new lesion formation and functional impairment.[22–25] Patients with active superficial circumscribed morphea may be treated with topical therapy or localized phototherapy.[24,25] Patients with active superficial generalized morphea may be treated with topical therapy, phototherapy, or a combination of systemic steroids and methotrexate based on patient preference and comorbidities.[24,25] Patients with morphea should also be counseled that treatment is not always necessary, particularly for asymptomatic disease that is not causing or at risk of causing functional limitations. Patients with morphea in the nonactive phase should be educated on signs of disease recurrence and offered clinical monitoring.

Lastly, but perhaps most importantly, patients need to leave their dermatologist's office understanding that morphea is not systemic sclerosis and will not increase their chances of developing systemic sclerosis in the future. Patient educational materials on morphea may be found through the *Journal of the American Medical Association Dermatology*.[26]

Morphea: estimate current practice

The MRA has surveyed the Medical Dermatology Society and Rheumatologic Dermatology Society on their current practices in regard to the evaluation and treatment of morphea (unpublished data). History, physical examination, and referrals to physical therapy and occupational therapy were regularly performed. Most respondents ordered autoantibodies in the evaluation of morphea, particularly anti-Scl70 and anticentromere antibodies (antibodies specific for systemic sclerosis). Respondents did not routinely have an organized and objective way of monitoring disease activity and response to therapy. Topical steroids are being routinely prescribed for subtypes of morphea that are unlikely to respond to topical therapy (linear disease, deep generalized disease). Methotrexate is not routinely prescribed for those patients with active linear morphea.

Additionally, it is estimated that very few clinicians assess the quality of life in their patients with morphea, perform examinations of the oral and genital mucosa,[27] rigorously assess for range-of-motion limitations, or educate patients on the difference between morphea and systemic sclerosis. Patients in the damage (ie, nonactive) phase of morphea may also be unnecessarily treated with immunosuppressants.

Morphea gaps

The gaps that exist in the care of patients with morphea result from lack of knowledge, specific practice patterns, the need for development of new skills, and the need for a change in attitudes. Development of defined best practices and guidelines for the evaluation and treatment of patients with morphea would help to close many of our knowledge, skill, specific practice, and attitude gaps. The lack of defined best practices contributes to the overuse of laboratory testing for autoantibodies, the lack of patient education on the differences between morphea and systemic sclerosis,

the lack of objective disease monitoring, the lack of aggressive treatment of morphea that impairs quality of life and physical functioning, the lack of quantification of quality-of-life issues in clinical practice, the lack of oral and genital mucosal examination to exclude mucosal involvement, and the inappropriate treatment of patients with morphea in the damage phase with immunosuppressant medications.

There are many barriers to developing best practices. The first step in developing guidelines for the assessment and treatment of a condition is to describe the current practices. Revealing how physicians are treating a rare condition to other physicians establishes treatment norms and, therefore, consensus. Consensus can then be used to establish guidelines. When studying rare diseases, data need to be pooled across practices in a standardized fashion to enable comparative effectiveness studies, which can then be used to establish best practices. Establishing best practices for a rare disease requires an international effort, a lot of protected time, and funding.

BEST PRACTICES IN MEDICAL EDUCATION

Residents are adult learners. Evidence has shown that adults learn best when the learning experience is interactive, is pertinent to the skills they need to acquire to best perform their jobs, allows for the ability to practice the skills that they learn, and provides constructive feedback on their performance.[28] Additional research on the science of learning has elucidated several strategies for learners and educators to use to maximize knowledge acquisition and application. These strategies include testing and retesting,[29,30] interspersed practice and spaced retrieval,[30–32] reflection and metacognition,[33–36] providing and receiving corrective feedback,[28,37] and cultivating a growth mindset.[38]

Best practices in educating our residents on the diagnosis and management of dermatomyositis, CLE, and morphea rely on involving residents in multidisciplinary and subspecialty clinics devoted to the care of patients with these relatively rare conditions. Knowledge retention is increased by making residents an integral team member in the evaluation and treatment of these patients and an active participant in their learning. Residents should be involved in reviewing outside records, compiling outside clinical data, interviewing and examining patients, efficiently presenting patients by including pertinent information and leaving out extraneous information, and developing a differential diagnosis with supporting and refuting facts for each diagnosis. Before presenting patients, the resident should also develop a plan for additional workup with reasoning as to why each test is important and how it will impact care, develop a plan for treatment with reasoning as to why 2 to 3 additional treatment options are less desirable, develop a plan for monitoring for medication toxicities, and deciding on an appropriate follow-up interval. If knowledge or skill gaps are revealed during a patient encounter, the resident should be involved in developing a plan for the acquisition of any knowledge or skill that was lacking. Knowledge retention is also increased by taking time at the end of clinic to reflect with the residents on what went well, what they can improve on, and their plan for improvement.

Ideally residents would rotate through multiple subspecialty clinics over months (ie, specific days assigned for each subspecialty clinic over months, instead of working in one subspecialty clinic for 1 month) to increase spaced retrieval. Studies have shown that massed practice (ie, rotating within the same subspecialty clinic for a month) increases the *perception* of knowledge gained but that spaced retrieval (ie, rotating in a subspecialty clinic 1 day a week over a long period of time) increases the actual knowledge gained.[31,32]

Before didactic sessions, educational materials should be shared with learners to help them to prepare for the session. Didactic sessions on DM, CLE, and morphea should start with pretests, include interactive cases that allow for dialogue and working through problems, and a posttest.

Estimate Current Practice

Most resident education occurs during clinical encounters and didactics. Clinical teaching tools, such as the 1-minute preceptor and reflective questioning, are likely not used with regularity. Feedback on resident performance in clinic may be infrequent or inadequate.[39,40] Residents and faculty may approach clinical reasoning with an entity theory (ie, thinking that intelligence and the ability to clinically reason is a fixed characteristic) and not with a growth mindset (ie, realizing that knowledge and clinical reasoning improve with effort and practice), limiting knowledge acquisition and growth.[38] Didactics are generally hour-long, noninteractive sessions.

The gaps that exist in CLE, DM, and morphea resident education are largely rooted in knowledge, interpersonal communication, and professionalism. Resident education in the care of CLE, DM, and morphea is lacking in adult learning theory and effective corrective feedback. Additionally, the rarity of these conditions and the rarity of subspecialty clinics devoted to the care of these patients results in infrequent patient care opportunities for residents.

Strategies to increase the efficacy of teaching and learning about CLE, DM, and morphea include incorporating adult learning theory into medical education and increasing effective feedback. Faculty may need educational sessions through their program director, their local graduate medical education department, the American Academy of Dermatology, or the Accreditation Council for Graduate Education. Additionally, these resources may also be used by faculty to sharpen feedback skills. Residents may be afforded the opportunity to rotate at centers with dedicated subspecialty clinics or offered rotations with other medical specialists who care for these patients. Simulated patients and on-line teaching may be an avenue to increase exposure to these conditions over time (ie, increasing delayed retrieval). Lastly, an increase awareness of combined internal medicine-dermatology training and medicine-dermatology fellowships may create more experts in these fields to teach in dermatology at academic centers.

REFERENCES

1. Albrecht J, Taylor L, Berlin JA, et al. The CLASI (Cutaneous LE Disease Area and Severity Index): an outcome instrument for cutaneous lupus erythematosus. J Invest Dermatol 2005;125:889–94.
2. Okon LG, Werth VP. Cutaneous lupus erythematosus: diagnosis and treatment. Best Pract Res Clin Rheumatol 2013;27:391–404.
3. Browning DJ. Impact of the revised American Academy of Ophthalmology guidelines regarding hydroxychloroquine screening on actual practice. Am J Ophthalmol 2013;155:418–28.e1.
4. A randomized study of the effect of withdrawing hydroxychloroquine sulfate in systemic lupus erythematosus. The Canadian Hydroxychloroquine Study Group. N Engl J Med 1991;324:150–4.
5. Mosca M, Tani C, Aringer M, et al. EULAR recommendations for monitoring systemic lupus erythematosus patients in clinical practice and in observational studies. Ann Rheum Dis 2010;69:1269–74.
6. Privette ED, Werth VP. Update on pathogenesis and treatment of CLE. Curr Opin Rheumatol 2013;25:584–90.
7. Kuhn A, Ruland V, Bonsmann G. Cutaneous lupus erythematosus: update of therapeutic options part II. J Am Acad Dermatol 2011;65:e195–213.
8. Kuhn A, Ruland V, Bonsmann G. Cutaneous lupus erythematosus: update of therapeutic options part I. J Am Acad Dermatol 2011;65:e179–93.
9. Chang AY, Ghazi E, Okawa J, et al. Quality of life differences between responders and nonresponders

in the treatment of cutaneous lupus erythematosus. JAMA Dermatol 2013;149:104–6.

10. Chang AY, Piette EW, Foering KP, et al. Response to antimalarials in cutaneous lupus erythematosus: a prospective analysis. Arch Dermatol 2011;147:1261–7.

11. Cortes-Hernandez J, Avila G, Vilardell-Tarres M, et al. Efficacy and safety of lenalidomide for refractory cutaneous lupus erythematosus. Arthritis Res Ther 2013;14:R265.

12. Okon L, Rosenbach M, Krathen M, et al. Lenalidomide in treatment-refractory cutaneous lupus erythematosus: efficacy and safety in a 52-week trial. J Am Acad Dermatol 2014;70:583–4.

13. Smith ES, Hallman JR, DeLuca AM, et al. Dermatomyositis: a clinicopathological study of 40 patients. Am J Dermatopathol 2009;31:61–7.

14. Tansley SL, Betteridge ZE, McHugh NJ. The diagnostic utility of autoantibodies in adult and juvenile myositis. Curr Opin Rheumatol 2013;25:772–7.

15. Lu X, Yang H, Shu X, et al. Factors predicting malignancy in patients with polymyositis and dermatomyositis: a systematic review and meta-analysis. PLoS One 2014;9:e94128.

16. Yassaee M, Fiorentino D, Taylor L, et al. Modification of the Cutaneous Dermatomyositis Disease Area and Severity Index, an outcome measure instrument. Br J Dermatol 2010;162:669–73.

17. Li SC, Torok KS, Pope E, et al. Development of consensus treatment plans for juvenile localized scleroderma: a roadmap toward comparative effectiveness studies in juvenile localized scleroderma. Arthritis Care Res (Hoboken) 2012;64:1175–85.

18. Laxer RM, Zulian F. Localized scleroderma. Curr Opin Rheumatol 2006;18:606–13.

19. Arkachaisri T, Vilaiyuk S, Li S, et al. The localized scleroderma skin severity index and physician global assessment of disease activity: a work in progress toward development of localized scleroderma outcome measures. J Rheumatol 2009;36:2819–29.

20. Zannin ME, Martini G, Athreya BH, et al. Ocular involvement in children with localised scleroderma: a multi-centre study. Br J Ophthalmol 2007;91:1311–4.

21. Chiu YE, Vora S, Kwon EK, et al. A significant proportion of children with morphea en coup de sabre and Parry-Romberg syndrome have neuroimaging findings. Pediatr Dermatol 2012;29:738–48.

22. Zulian F, Vallongo C, Patrizi A, et al. A long-term follow-up study of methotrexate in juvenile localized scleroderma (morphea). J Am Acad Dermatol 2012;67:1151–6.

23. Zulian F, Martini G, Vallongo C, et al. Methotrexate treatment in juvenile localized scleroderma: a randomized, double-blind, placebo-controlled trial. Arthritis Rheum 2011;63:1998–2006.

24. Fett N, Werth VP. Update on morphea: part II. Outcome measures and treatment. J Am Acad Dermatol 2011;64:231–42 [quiz: 243–4].

25. Zwischenberger BA, Jacobe HT. A systematic review of morphea treatments and therapeutic algorithm. J Am Acad Dermatol 2011;65:925–41.

26. Fett NM. Morphea (localized scleroderma). JAMA Dermatol 2013;149:1124.

27. Lutz V, Frances C, Bessis D, et al. High frequency of genital lichen sclerosus in a prospective series of 76 patients with morphea: toward a better understanding of the spectrum of morphea. Arch Dermatol 2012;148:24–8.

28. Reed S, Shell R, Kassis K, et al. Applying adult learning practices in medical education. Curr Probl Pediatr Adolesc Health Care 2014;44:170–81.

29. McDaniel MA, Bugg JM, Liu Y, et al. When does the test-study-test sequence optimize learning and retention? J Exp Psychol Appl 2015;21:370–82.

30. McCabe J. Metacognitive awareness of learning strategies in undergraduates. Mem Cognit 2011;39:462–76.

31. Karpicke JD, Bauernschmidt A. Spaced retrieval: absolute spacing enhances learning regardless of relative spacing. J Exp Psychol Learn Mem Cogn 2011;37:1250–7.

32. Karpicke JD, Roediger HL 3rd. Expanding retrieval practice promotes short-term retention, but equally spaced retrieval enhances long-term retention. J Exp Psychol Learn Mem Cogn 2007;33:704–19.

33. Ibiapina C, Mamede S, Moura A, et al. Effects of free, cued and modelled reflection on medical students' diagnostic competence. Med Educ 2014;48:796–805.

34. Mamede S, Schmidt HG. Reflection in diagnostic reasoning: what really matters? Acad Med 2014;89:959–60.

35. Mamede S, van Gog T, Moura AS, et al. Reflection as a strategy to foster medical students' acquisition of diagnostic competence. Med Educ 2012;46:464–72.

36. Mamede S, van Gog T, Sampaio AM, et al. How can students' diagnostic competence benefit most from practice with clinical cases? The effects of structured reflection on future diagnosis of the same and novel diseases. Acad Med 2014;89:121–7.

37. Mayer RE. Applying the science of learning to medical education. Med Educ 2010;44:543–9.

38. Teunissen PW, Bok HG. Believing is seeing: how people's beliefs influence goals, emotions and behaviour. Med Educ 2013;47:1064–72.

39. Hewson MG, Little ML. Giving feedback in medical education: verification of recommended techniques. J Gen Intern Med 1998;13:111–6.

40. Branch WT Jr, Paranjape A. Feedback and reflection: teaching methods for clinical settings. Acad Med 2002;77:1185–8.

Practice and Educational Gaps in Blistering Disease

Nazanin Ehsani-Chimeh, MD[a], M. Peter Marinkovich, MD[a,b],*

KEYWORDS

• Blistering • Bullous • Autoimmunity • Pemphigus • Pemphigoid

KEY POINTS

- Autoimmune bullous patients often remain either undiagnosed for prolonged periods of time or poorly diagnosed without immunologic confirmation, resulting in significant additional morbidity.
- The most important principle in management of autoimmune bullous disease is to halt blistering activity while minimizing side effects of medications especially corticosteroids.
- Judicious use of systemic steroids and steroid-sparing agents are essential tools in the management of autoimmune bullous disease patients.
- Rituximab and intravenous immunoglobulin are playing increasingly important and earlier roles in the management of many autoimmune bullous patients.
- Understanding of and surveillance for drug side effects are critical in the long-term management of the autoimmune bullous patient.

DIAGNOSTIC POINTS

Diagnosis is a critical first step in the care of autoimmune bullous disease patients. It is, unfortunately, all too common for a patient to go for many months, or even years, until the correct diagnosis is finally made.[1] Excess suffering due to the painful blisters and erosions of pemphigus, or the intractable itching of pemphigoid is only part of the costs paid to delayed diagnosis. During this undiagnosed period, the patients are usually empirically given high-dose systemic steroids. This incurs its share of the cumulative morbidity. Another factor to consider in late diagnosis is the degree of chronicity it evokes on the disease phenotype. Most dermatologists can appreciate that it is often the case that the more chronic a skin condition becomes, the longer and more difficult it is to eradicate. In the instance of poorly treated autoimmune bullous disease, this may translate into increased development of a B cell memory compartment promoting the chronic production of pathologic antibodies, which may become more difficult to eradicate with specific therapies such as rituximab[2] once the diagnosis is finally made.

In addition to delay of diagnosis, another common problem is the assumption of a diagnosis based on clinical and histologic examination only. Well-intentioned dermatopathologists, whose histologic observations "suggestive of" or "consistent with" some type of autoimmune bullous disease, are too often taken by clinicians as proof of a given diagnosis, without further testing. This can be a great disservice for patients.

Consider the case of a patient with a putative diagnosis of bullous pemphigoid, based on histology and clinical appearance alone, without immunologic confirmation. After high-dose corticosteroid therapy for many months or even years, this cushingoid patient presents to the clinician's office, who immediately performs a direct immunofluorescence

Disclosure Statement: The authors have nothing to disclose.
a Department of Dermatology, Stanford University School of Medicine, 269 Campus Drive, CCSR Building, Room 2145, Stanford, CA 94305-5168, USA; b Veterans Administration Medical Center, Palo Alto, CA, USA
* Corresponding author.
E-mail address: mpm@stanford.edu

Dermatol Clin 34 (2016) 251–256
http://dx.doi.org/10.1016/j.det.2016.02.001
0733-8635/16/$ – see front matter Published by Elsevier Inc.

derm.theclinics.com

(DIF) biopsy and demonstrates linear immunoglobulin (Ig)A disease, which can look clinically and histologically identical to bullous pemphigoid. After dapsone therapy is initiated and the patient completely weaned off prednisone with excellent disease control, the clinician realizes that if prompt immunologic testing had been performed, prolonged high-dose steroid use and all the concomitant morbidity could have been avoided. This example is just 1 of many demonstrating why an immunologic diagnosis is so essential for these patients.

The choices of immunologic tests available for correctly diagnosing immunobullous diseases are numerous. In addition to perilesional DIF microscopy biopsy (the most sensitive test), serum from patients with active disease can be analyzed by indirect immunofluorescence (IIF). More recently, enzyme-linked immunosorbent assay (ELISA) assays are also used. It is not just for desmogleins 1 and 3, but it is also now available for bullous pemphigoid and epidermolysis bullosa acquisita (EBA) antigens.

With a positive DIF or high enough titer IIF or ELISA, any of these are sufficient to make the correct diagnosis. One key point is that these tests should be performed while the patient is showing disease activity. It is suboptimal to perform these tests after the patient has been placed on high-dose immunosuppressive therapy. A diminution of the immune response from such high-dose therapy could lead to a false-negative result. For this reason, it is important to plan ahead and look to perform the immunologic diagnosis early before systemic therapy is implemented.

False-negative results can also be a result of lesional, as opposed to perilesional, DIF biopsies or because DIF biopsies are inadvertently placed in a medium other than Michel's or Zeus medium. Biopsies that sit around for too long while one is trying to obtain the proper medium, or sera that is not promptly sent out to the appropriate laboratory, are also very likely to result in false-negative results. It is, therefore, critical to plan ahead, obtain the proper holding medium in advance, and communicate with the testing laboratories as well as clinic staff to make sure transfer of specimens for immunologic testing is carried out correctly and expeditiously.

These examples illustrate that it is important to look at negative immunologic results in suspected autoimmune bullous patients with a skeptical eye. Were the biopsies correctly performed? Was the serum correctly analyzed? Was the patient tested at a time when the disease was active? These are the questions that should come to mind when analyzing negative immunologic test results.

Based on experience with the above variables, it is clear that 1 negative immunologic result does not necessarily rule out the diagnosis. Therefore, if the patient continues to display characteristic features of autoimmune bullous diseases, it is important to consider repeat testing of previously negative results, especially during periods of high disease activity.

Another difficulty sometimes encountered in subepidermal autoimmune bullous diagnosis is in distinguishing among the individual subtypes. For example, EBA can sometimes histologically and clinically mimic either cicatricial or bullous pemphigoid. However, these diseases can differ in their prognosis and response to therapy. In addition, there is a subtype of cicatricial pemphigoid characterized by antibodies against laminin-332 (sometimes still referred to by its previous name epiligrin). This antilaminin-332 form of cicatricial pemphigoid has an increased association with (and can sometimes precede) the development of a variety of different types of cancers.[3] It is important, therefore, to correctly determine which of these subepidermal diseases the autoimmune patient has and this requires specialized evaluation of the dermal-epidermal basement membrane (BMZ).

Common belief is that periodic acid–Schiff–diastase stain permits visualization of the BMZ; however, what is in fact visualized is a precipitation of dye many times the thickness of the actual BMZ.[4] In fact, at approximately 0.2 μm in thickness, the dermal-epidermal BMZ is well below the resolution of light microscopy. However, a useful light microscopy–based tool has been developed to circumvent this limitation. Skin samples incubated in 1 M sodium chloride will eventually separate in the center of the BMZ, in a region known as the lamina lucida.[5,6] Above the lamina lucida in the epidermal roof of salt-split skin lies the bullous pemphigoid antigens, as well as other less commonly encountered antigens such as β4 integrin, targeted in some forms of cicatricial pemphigoid. Other antigens, such as type VII collagen (the EBA antigen) and laminin-332 localize to the dermal side of the salt-induced split.

Therefore salt-split skin analysis has the ability to distinguish bullous pemphigoid and many forms of cicatricial pemphigoid, in which immunoreactants would mainly localize to the epidermal roof of the split from EBA, and the laminin-332 subtype of cicatricial pemphigoid, in which immunoreactants would localize to the dermal floor of the split. This type of salt-split skin analysis can be performed on DIF as well as IIF samples, depending on the capabilities of the laboratory. Thus, when one suspects a subepidermal bullous skin disease, it makes sense to perform salt-split skin DIF or IIF analysis instead of conventional DIF or IIF analysis.

The availability of ELISA assays in recent years is of great utility in the subclassification of the subepidermal bullous diseases. By distinguishing between autoantibody reactivity with the bullous pemphigoid antigens compared with type VII collagen, these ELISA tests can be quite helpful as an alternative to salt-split skin analysis. However, as of this writing, an ELISA test is not yet widely available for laminin-332 because it is a difficult protein to manufacture. Therefore, only a handful of specialized laboratories are currently able to perform laminin-332 antibody analysis.

THERAPEUTIC POINTS

A great deal of overlap exists between the treatment of patients with subepidermal and intraepidermal bullous diseases; however, an important distinction is the clinical response to topical therapy. The basis of these differences is illustrated in animal models. These models have shown that pemphigus antibodies are themselves pathogenic,[7,8] whereas pemphigoid antibodies show a greater reliance on complement fixation and the participation of local immune cells in the skin for blistering activity.[9] Because topical therapy is not going to significantly decrease total circulating antibodies, it is not going to benefit pemphigus patients as well as it is going to benefit patients with subepidermal bullous disorders such as pemphigoid. Therefore, bullous pemphigoid therapy is enhanced with a component of topical therapy, either as a sole agent or in combination with systemic therapy.[10] Bullous pemphigoid also responds to the combination of tetracyclines and niacinamide.[11,12] In pemphigoid patients not responding to these milder therapies, and in pemphigus patients who usually do not respond well to these milder therapies, a systemic immunosuppressive approach is usually needed.[13]

Before the onset of corticosteroids, pemphigus was often a fatal disease. Corticosteroids still remain the most widely used class of drugs for all patients with IgG-mediated autoimmune bullous disease (see later discussion of IgA patients and use of dapsone). For severe patients, systemic corticosteroids such as prednisone are essential in bringing a halt to new blistering disease activity. This halt, which is sometimes referred to as capturing the disease, is a critical first step in controlling a severe flare. Failure to halt new blistering disease activity in a severe flare will usually thwart all subsequent therapeutic attempts, allowing the disease process to smolder

along until it eventually reflares. Usually, 1 mg per kilogram of prednisone is sufficient to halt such flares but sometimes higher doses are needed.

Once the new blistering disease activity is halted in severe cases, then the focus of therapy is to minimize the total amount of systemic steroids over the long term to reduce associated morbidity. Minimizing this morbidity is optimized by a judicious use of prednisone as well as the timely use of steroid-sparing agents. As blistering disease activity is halted, the natural tendency is to try to taper the steroids as quickly as possible. However, lowering too quickly can be highly problematic due to the tendency of the disease process to rebound. Another common misuse of systemic steroids in these patients is through the use of intramuscular or subcutaneous steroid injections. In either case, steroid effects wear off too fast and, as a result, the patient's disease activity rebounds, either back to the original level or even higher. Thus, lowering prednisone more slowly to avoid rebound flares may reduce the total prednisone burden in the long term.

Once the disease is fully stabilized, an initial taper of prednisone at a rate of 10 mg per day each week, is practical. However, it is important to taper systemic steroids more slowly once the level of 40 mg per day is reached. One approach is to lower by 1 mg a day every 2 days. Another approach is to taper by 1 mg every other day. The latter is useful in that it brings the patient down to 40 mg every other day. After this, tapering can take place by 1 mg every other day with the goal of getting below 20 mg every other day. This is beneficial in that every other day prednisone therapy may have fewer side effects compared with every day prednisone.[14] Once at the level of 10 mg per day or 20 mg every other day, the long term effects are much less.

With this slow-tapering regimen, a major flare during the tapering process is less likely. However, during the taper, both the patient and physician should remain vigilant in watching for the return of new disease activity. If any activity is noted, the tapering should be put on hold. Often with this slow of a prednisone taper, new disease activity, if it does come up, will be mild and will subside after a week or 2. At this point, the taper can be carefully resumed. If the disease activity does not subside or worsens, it is important to act quickly to stop the flare. In this regard, it is important for the blistering disease patient to have close communication with the treating physician so that flares can be promptly reported. A general rule of thumb is that if a significant flare does occur during the tapering process, prednisone should be increased by 50% immediately to capture the disease activity. It is this principle of slow tapering and rapid increase that is essential in the judicious management of systemic steroids in autoimmune bullous patients.

In addition to proper tapering of systemic steroids, an important management principle is the effective use of steroid-sparing agents.[15] Two first-line steroid-sparing agents, azathioprine and mycophenolic acid, act similarly by reducing the humoral immune response, with the former having greater hepatotoxicity and the latter being more expensive. Cyclophosphamide is another alternative, which is more effective than azathioprine or mycophenolic acid; however, it is more toxic. If it is suspected that systemic steroids cannot be tapered to below the equivalent of 10 mg per day prednisone, it is important to implement 1 of these steroid-sparing agents early.

An important consideration in comanagement of steroid-sparing agents and prednisone is coordination of the tapering process once disease activity is stabilized. Two important principles are (1) do not taper 2 therapies at the same time and (2) taper the most toxic therapy first. Considering the relative toxicity of steroid-sparing agents and systemic steroids, it is generally agreed that high-dose steroids are more toxic than steroid-sparing agents. However, it is debatable whether prednisone at less than 10 mg a day is more or less toxic than steroid-sparing agents. One approach is to taper steroids completely off and subsequently work on tapering the steroid-sparing agent. Another approach is to taper prednisone to less than 10 mg a day, then pause the prednisone taper and work instead on tapering the steroid-sparing agents. Then, once the steroid-sparing agents are tapered off, to go back to tapering the last amount of prednisone.

One of the limitations of the former approach is that it requires managing autoimmune bullous disease with steroid-sparing agents alone. This is problematic due to the typically slow response the steroid-sparing agents often have. It normally takes about 3 to 4 weeks to see the effects of steroid-sparing agent, compared with prednisone, which produces effects in the patient disease course within several days. Autoimmune bullous diseases are dynamic processes and require precise shifts of therapy in response to rising or lowering disease activity. Using steroid-sparing agents to do this is somewhat akin to driving an ocean liner, in which a turn of the wheel might take several miles before showing an effect. In contrast, using low-dose prednisone therapy to treat residual disease is like driving a sports car, with a nimble response seen in the disease activity

immediately following a turn of the wheel. For this reason, it seems practical in the later stages of disease management to taper off the steroid-sparing agent first, and then to go back to managing the patients residual activity with low-dose prednisone.

It may be necessary to go beyond conventional steroid-sparing agents to more advanced agents such as rituximab and intravenous immunoglobulin. These agents should be carefully considered if disease activity does not permit tapering of prednisone to less than 10 mg a day, or allow tapering off of steroid-sparing agents. These advanced agents are the most obviously useful in severe cases in which prednisone cannot be brought down from high levels. However, there are a subset of patients whose disease is less severe, but none-the-less stubborn, and whose steroid requirements are more moderate but persistent over many years. In these patients, it is important to consider the long-term toxicity of even moderate steroid therapy. In these moderate but recalcitrant patients, advanced therapies such as rituximab or intravenous immunoglobulin should also be considered.

A recently emerging question is whether rituximab or intravenous immunoglobulin should be considered tertiary, secondary, or first-line therapy.[16] In the instance of rituximab, several studies, including large studies in France, have demonstrated the effectiveness of rituximab compared with conventional steroid-sparing agents. Intravenous immunoglobulin, with its nonimmunosuppressive toxicity profile, can be especially useful in patients at increased risk for infections. For all these reasons, the autoimmune bullous field may be shifting to earlier use of each of these infusion-based therapies in the future. In anticipation of this shift, it will be important to emphasize management of infusion therapies in current dermatology residency programs. In managing patients, it is essential to know the appropriate infusion protocols, premedications, as-needed medication dosing, and how to form a close working relationship with infusion staff, to be able to respond quickly and effectively to infusion reactions when they arise.

Dapsone is a drug which has been in the dermatologist's arsenal for some time and can be highly effective for IgA-mediated bullous diseases, especially linear IgA disease[17] and dermatitis herpetiformis, as well as some cases of EBA. Although it typically is of more limited benefit in the treatment of pemphigus or pemphigoid, it can often substitute for low-dose prednisone in these patients. It can be especially useful in pemphigus and pemphigoid patients with exacerbating comorbidities such as diabetes.

Despite its obvious usefulness, there is sometimes a tendency to use dapsone hesitantly or without a full therapeutic trial. Some clinicians seem reluctant to go beyond a certain dose, such as 75 or 100 mg a day. Because the maximum tolerated dapsone dose varies considerably from patient to patient, it is important that each patient be treated individually. A rational approach to using dapsone in nonanemic patients who have no contraindicating comorbidities is to obtain a glucose 6 phosphate dehydrogenase level, and a complete blood count (CBC). If these are satisfactory, one can start at a low dose, such as 25 mg a day, which can be incrementally increased by 25 mg a day each week, in concert with weekly CBC blood tests to look for hemolysis. Then the dose can be increased until disease efficacy is noticed. If during this course, the hemoglobin drops by 1 g but not more than 2 g without disease improvement, the therapeutic trial can be considered unsuccessful.

One point that is often discussed but which nonetheless deserves emphasis is the need to monitor for cumulative side effects of medications. In patients on long-term corticosteroids, monitoring for the development of secondary osteoporosis and managing with bisphosphonates, as well as calcium and vitamin D supplements is important. Patients on long-term corticosteroids also should be screened regularly by an ophthalmologist for development of cataracts or glaucoma, as well as monitored for development of diabetes and hypertension by their primary care physicians. Patients on dapsone should be observed for the rare but significant dapsone hypersensitivity syndrome but also should be followed for more long-term symptoms of hemolysis, methemoglobinemia, and peripheral neuropathy. Side effects of steroid-sparing agents (eg, azathioprine and mycophenolic acid), such as cytopenia and hepatic inflammation, should be carefully looked for and, in the case of cyclophosphamide, copious hydration of the patient and intermittent monitoring of the urine is extremely helpful to address the serious complication of hematuria. Beyond these most-obvious examples of drug toxicities, it behooves the bullous disease practitioner to know in detail the less common side effects of all of these agents and to be ready to provide detailed information to patients and consulting physicians.

Finally, in the management of autoimmune bullous patients there is an important need for a multidisciplinary approach. For example, in patients with significant oral disease, an oral medicine specialist can be extremely helpful in managing oral care and in coordinating topical oral therapy (eg, construction of dental trays to hold topical corticosteroids in the treatment of gingival disease). Similarly, in patients with vulvar or vaginal mucosal disease, a gynecologist familiar with autoimmune bullous disease can be extremely helpful. In patients with cicatricial pemphigoid or EBA involving the oropharynx or eyes, an ears, nose, and throat specialist or ophthalmologist is essential in assessing disease activity as an aid in gauging therapies. To help prevent development of diabetes or other complications of long-term steroid use, an endocrinologist can play an essential role in disease management. Last, but not least, the bullous disease specialist needs to coordinate closely with the patient's primary care doctor in the overall care plan.

In summary, care of patients with autoimmune bullous disease can be quite challenging. However, with patience and determined efforts, these diseases can and often do resolve and go into remission. This knowledge offers hope to the patient and is an essential goal to strive toward for the treating physician.

REFERENCES

1. Zillikens D. Diagnosis of autoimmune bullous skin diseases. Clin Lab 2008;54:491–503.
2. Colliou N, Picard D, Caillot F, et al. Long-term remissions of severe pemphigus after rituximab therapy are associated with prolonged failure of desmoglein B cell response. Sci Transl Med 2013;5:175ra130.
3. Egan CA, Lazarova Z, Darling TN, et al. Anti-epiligrin cicatricial pemphigoid: clinical findings, immunopathogenesis, and significant associations. Medicine (Baltimore) 2003;82:177–86.
4. Briggaman RA, Wheeler CE. The epidermal-dermal junction. J Invest Dermatol 1975;65:71–84.
5. Lazarova Z, Yancey KB. Reactivity of autoantibodies from patients with defined subepidermal bullous diseases against 1 mol/L salt-split skin. Specificity, sensitivity, and practical considerations. J Am Acad Dermatol 1996;35:398–403.
6. Gammon WR, Fine JD, Forbes M, et al. Immunofluorescence on salt-split skin for the detection and differentiation of BMZ autoantibodies. J Am Acad Dermatol 1992;27:79–87.
7. Anhalt GJ, Diaz LA. Pemphigus vulgaris—a model for cutaneous autoimmunity. J Am Acad Dermatol 2004;51:S20–1.
8. Grando SA. Pemphigus autoimmunity: hypotheses and realities. Autoimmunity 2012;45:7–35.
9. Liu Z, Sui W, Zhao M, et al. Subepidermal blistering induced by human autoantibodies to BP180 requires innate immune players in a humanized bullous pemphigoid mouse model. J Autoimmun 2008;31:331–8.

10. Schmidt E, Zillikens D. Pemphigoid diseases. Lancet 2013;381:320–32.

11. Hornschuh B, Hamm H, Wever S, et al. Treatment of 16 patients with bullous pemphigoid with oral tetracycline and niacinamide and topical clobetasol. J Am Acad Dermatol 1997;36:101–3.

12. Kolbach DN, Remme JJ, Bos WH, et al. Bullous pemphigoid successfully controlled by tetracycline and nicotinamide. Br J Dermatol 1995;133:88–90.

13. Santoro FA, Stoopler ET, Werth VP. Pemphigus. Dent Clin North Am 2013;57:597–610.

14. Gluck OS, Murphy WA, Hahn TJ, et al. Bone loss in adults receiving alternate day glucocorticoid therapy. A comparison with daily therapy. Arthritis Rheum 1981;24(7):892–8.

15. Atzmony L, Hodak E, Leshem YA, et al. The role of adjuvant therapy in pemphigus: a systematic review and meta-analysis. J Am Acad Dermatol 2015;73: 264–71.

16. Ingen-Housz-Oro S, Valeyrie-Allanore L, Cosnes A, et al. First-line treatment of pemphigus vulgaris with a combination of rituximab and high-potency topical corticosteroids. JAMA Dermatol 2015;151: 200–3.

17. Fortuna G, Marinkovich MP. Linear immunoglobulin A bullous dermatosis. Clin Dermatol 2012;30:38–50.

Practice Gaps in Pruritus

Jonathan I. Silverberg, MD, PhD, MPH[a,b,c,d],*

KEYWORDS

• Itch • Pruritus • Assessment • Treatment • Workup • Education

KEY POINTS

- The severity of and patient-burden from pruritus should be assessed in all patients with itch.
- Management of pruritus should be tailored to the underlying cause and use evidence-based treatments.
- Patients with generalized pruritus of nondermatologic cause should be screened for several underlying systemic disorders.

PRACTICE GAPS

Difficulty Measuring Pruritus

Pruritus or itch is a sensation that is characterized by an urge to scratch. Patients' report of pruritus is subjective and can be described as itching, burning, tingling, stinging, and so forth. Given the subjective nature of pruritus, it is often difficult to assess in clinical practice. There are currently no serologic or tissue markers clinically available to characterize the nature and/or intensity of itch (**Box 1**). In order to address this knowledge and skill gap, future studies are needed to identify biomarkers of itch that can be used in clinical practice. One approach to objectively assessing itch is to measure body movements that occur in scratching (ie, actigraphy). This approach has been used in research studies and clinical trials. However, the feasibility and validity of using actigraphy in clinical practice has not been established. Future studies are needed to determine whether actigraphy should have a role in clinical practice.

Clinical assessment of pruritus is currently limited to patient-reported outcomes, including the visual analog scale (VAS) and numeric rating scale (NRS). These tools have been previously validated.[1] Some experts have even suggested incorporating such measures of itch as a fifth vital sign in dermatology practice, similar to the routine use of similar scales for the assessment of pain. However, these scores are imperfect. Self-reported intensity of itch with VAS seems to not correlate well with objective measures of scratching using actigraphy.[2] Nevertheless, until optimal objective measures for itch are available for clinical practice, the VAS or NRS remain important tools for quantifying the intensity of itch. Alternatively, the patient-burden of itch on can be assessed using quality-of-life instruments (eg, Dermatology Life Quality Index, Skindex, or ItchyQOL). Unfortunately, standardized assessment of itch is rarely performed in dermatological practice outside of specialty centers. In order to address this practice gap, health care professionals in dermatology should consider routine screening of patients for

Financial Disclosures: None.

Conflicts of Interest: None.

Funding Support: This publication was made possible with support from the Agency for Healthcare Research and Quality (AHRQ), grant number K12HS023011, and the Dermatology Foundation.

[a] Department of Dermatology, Northwestern University Feinberg School of Medicine, 676 North St. Clair Street, Suite 1600, Chicago, IL 60611, USA; [b] Department of Preventive Medicine, Northwestern University Feinberg School of Medicine, 676 North St. Clair Street, Suite 1600, Chicago, IL 60611, USA; [c] Department of Medical Social Sciences, Northwestern University Feinberg School of Medicine, 676 North St. Clair Street, Suite 1600, Chicago, IL 60611, USA; [d] Northwestern Medicine Multidisciplinary Eczema Center, 676 North St. Clair Street, Suite 1600, Chicago, IL 60611, USA

* Department of Dermatology, Northwestern University Feinberg School of Medicine, 676 North St. Clair Street, Suite 1600, Chicago, IL 60611, USA.

E-mail address: JonathanISilverberg@Gmail.com

Dermatol Clin 34 (2016) 257–261

http://dx.doi.org/10.1016/j.det.2016.02.008

Box 1
Practice gaps for the evaluation and management of itch

Practice gaps

   Difficulty measuring itch

- Lack of biomarkers for itch
- Lack of objective measures of itch available for clinical use
- Infrequent use of validated patient-reported measures of itch by health care professionals

   Lack of appreciation of the patient-burden of itch

   Limited treatment options for itch

- There are no FDA-approved medications primarily indicated for the treatment of itch.
- Dermatologists often use non–evidence-based treatments for itch and may not be comfortable with prescribing some of the more effective treatments available.
- Antihistamines should not be a one-size-fits-all treatment of all pruritic disorders.
- Screening and referral for mental health comorbidity of itch are often not performed.

   Lack of evidence for workup of generalized pruritus

- Generalized pruritus may be caused by several systemic disorders.
- There is no consensus for the optimal screening approach for systemic disease.

Educational gaps

   Many dermatologic texts do not have sections devoted to the evaluation and management of pruritus.

   Dermatology residency curricula should incorporate didactics devoted towards the evidence-based treatment of pruritus.

Abbreviation: FDA, Food and Drug Administration.

---

itch. At the very least, patients with chronic inflammatory skin disease or who present with a chief complaint of pruritus should be evaluated with VAS or NRS. Strategies to improve the clinical assessment of itch include incorporating the VAS or NRS into the electronic health record and incorporating itch assessments into the clinical workflow when patients are being roomed.

Lack of Appreciation of the Patient-Burden of Pruritus

Chronic pruritus is a very troubling symptom for patients and associated with poor health-related quality of life.[3,4] Previous studies found that itch causes just as much quality-of-life disturbance as does pain.[5] Chronic pruritus negatively effects all patients' activities of daily living and their emotional well-being.[3,4] Despite itch being a commonly reported symptom,[6] it is not routinely assessed by most clinicians. Patients often think that health professionals do not take their itch seriously,[7] which may result in inadequate treatment and poor patient satisfaction. To address these gaps, health care professionals should routinely ask patients about itch. Moreover, health care

professionals should ask patients with pruritus about its impact on their quality of life. Finally, treatment decisions must factor in the patient-burden of itch. Health care professionals should consider adding and/or replacing itch treatments when the intensity of itch and quality-of-life disturbance are not improved by current therapy.

Limited Treatment Options for Pruritus

There are several gaps with respect to the treatment of itch. There are no Food and Drug Administration–approved medications primarily indicated for the treatment of itch. The mechanisms of itch are not fully understood, which has hindered development of novel therapeutic agents for pruritus. Moreover, itch seems to be mediated by complex signals from both peripheral and central nervous system pathways. It remains controversial whether future therapeutic development should target peripheral or central pathways. Future research is needed in order to better understand both the peripheral and central mechanisms for itch.

Moreover, far fewer randomized controlled trials have been performed to study the efficacy of treatments for itch than for pain. More well-designed randomized controlled trials are needed to determine the most effective treatments for itch.

There are a variety of causes of itch, including inflammatory skin diseases (eg, atopic dermatitis and lichen planus), systemic disease (eg, renal or hepatic failure), burns, and so forth. Itch may respond differentially to treatment depending on the cause. For example, topical treatments are quite effective in chronic inflammatory skin disease but are not particularly effective for uremic pruritus. Over-the-counter antipruritic agents (eg, menthol) may not be effective for systemic causes of itch.[8] Ursodeoxycholic acid seems to be effective for the treatment of intrahepatic cholestasis of pregnancy.[9,10] Patients with uremic pruritus typically improve with improved renal function or dialysis. Thus, treatment of itch should be tailored to the cause.

Antihistamines are commonly used for the treatment of itch. Antihistamines may be effective for the treatment of itch secondary to urticaria,[11] which is a histamine-mediated disorder. Moreover, the sedating properties of first-generation antihistamines can be used to help pruritic patients fall asleep at night. However, antihistamines are generally ineffective treatments for the reduction of other types of itch. Moreover, high doses of antihistamines are associated with a variety of adverse effects, including daytime somnolence, weight gain, dry mouth, urinary retention, dizziness, and so forth. Although later-generation antihistamines have fewer adverse effects, they are also unlikely to be effective at reducing itch and do not have the sedating properties to help patients fall asleep. Therefore, antihistamines are not recommended for the treatment of itch in atopic dermatitis[12] and should not be a one-size-fits-all treatment of other pruritic disorders.

There are several existing therapies that should be used as first-line agents or considered as second-line agents if and when patients experience treatment failure with antihistamines. Gabapentin has been found to be effective in uremic pruritus,[13–15] burns,[16] notalgia paresthestica,[17] neuropathic itch,[14] and itch occurring in palliative patients.[13,18] Additional agents that should be considered for the treatment of itch include pregabalin, mirtazapine, butorphenone, naltrexone, aprepitant, and narrow-band ultraviolet B.[9,13,14,19–22] Of note, placebo effects on itch are common,[23] which may explain why some patients report improvement of their itch even with several non–evidence-based treatments. Nevertheless, health care professionals should use evidence-based treatments wherever possible.

Finally, patients with chronic pruritus often require psychological interventions as part of their treatment plan.[24] This requirement may be true regardless of the cause of itch. Many dermatologists do not ask patients about the impact of itch on their mental health. Understandably, most dermatologists are not skilled in administering appropriate psychological interventions. In addition, such interventions are time consuming and may not integrate into the clinical workflow of the typical dermatology practice. Nevertheless, health care professionals should consider a brief assessment of the impact of itch on mental health and refer to an appropriate mental health specialist for long-term treatment.

Lack of Evidence for Workup of Generalized Pruritus

Itch can be the first symptom of systemic disease, including uremia, cholestasis, thyroid disease, human immunodeficiency virus, polycythemia vera, diabetes, leukemia, and lymphoma, including Hodgkin disease, cutaneous T-cell lymphoma, and Sézary syndrome.[25] In addition, specific causes of itch may have an improved response to tailored treatment. Thus, it is imperative to evaluate pruritic patients for underlying systemic disorders. However, the myriad disorders that are associated with itch present a clinical challenge. There are no consensus guidelines as to the best algorithm for working up generalized pruritus. Comprehensive screening for all these disorders can be quite expensive. Moreover, the prevalence of these disorders is low in the general population, which results in infrequent positives and a low positive predictive value. Many patients with generalized pruritus have entirely negative blood work and imaging. Future research is needed to determine the optimal algorithm for evaluating systemic causes of generalized pruritus. Until then, health care practitioners should perform a comprehensive patient history, review of systems, and physical examination to identify clinical clues toward the cause of itch. Particular attention should be paid toward evidence of a skin disorder that might cause pruritus, including xerosis and visible inflammation of skin. If these are not present, then age-appropriate and, if needed, comprehensive screening for the various systemic causes of itch should be considered.

Dermatologists may not recognize the potential role of medications as an iatrogenic cause of itch. Medication use should be assessed in patients with generalized pruritus, because calcium channel blockers, hydrochlorothiazide, and other medications may cause itch without any other cutaneous findings.[26]

EDUCATIONAL GAPS

The etiopathogenesis and treatment of itch is complex. The workup of itch is challenging and requires a broad differential diagnosis. Residents must be fluent in the spectrum of possible causes, ranging from benign disorders (eg, xerosis and atopic dermatitis) to malignancy (eg, cutaneous T-cell lymphoma and paraneoplastic itch) and systemic disease (eg, uremia). Many dermatologic texts do not have sections devoted to the evaluation and management of pruritus. Dermatology residency curricula should incorporate didactics, particularly generalized pruritus.

Treatment of itch often requires the use of oral medications that are outside the comfort zone of dermatologists. These medications include neuroleptics, selective serotonin uptake inhibitors, benzodiazepines, immunosuppressants, and so forth. Many dermatology residents graduate from residency without learning how to when and how to administer these medications. It is vital that dermatology residency curricula incorporate didactics devoted toward the evidence-based treatment of pruritus, including an appropriate therapeutic ladder for different causes of itch.

REFERENCES

1. Phan NQ, Blome C, Fritz F, et al. Assessment of pruritus intensity: prospective study on validity and reliability of the visual analogue scale, numerical rating scale and verbal rating scale in 471 patients with chronic pruritus. Acta Derm Venereol 2012;92:502–7.
2. Murray CS, Rees JL. Are subjective accounts of itch to be relied on? The lack of relation between visual analogue itch scores and actigraphic measures of scratch. Acta Derm Venereol 2011;91:18–23.
3. Warlich B, Fritz F, Osada N, et al. Health-related quality of life in chronic pruritus: an analysis related to disease etiology, clinical skin conditions and itch intensity. Dermatology 2015;231:253–9.
4. Erturk IE, Arican O, Omurlu IK, et al. Effect of the pruritus on the quality of life: a preliminary study. Ann Dermatol 2012;24:406–12.
5. Kini SP, DeLong LK, Veledar E, et al. The impact of pruritus on quality of life: the skin equivalent of pain. Arch Dermatol 2011;147:1153–6.
6. Weisshaar E, Dalgard F. Epidemiology of itch: adding to the burden of skin morbidity. Acta Derm Venereol 2009;89:339–50.
7. Bathe A, Weisshaar E, Matterne U. Chronic pruritus–more than a symptom: a qualitative investigation into patients' subjective illness perceptions. J Adv Nurs 2013;69:316–26.
8. Krajnik M, Zylicz Z. Understanding pruritus in systemic disease. J Pain Symptom Manage 2001;21:151–68.
9. Pongcharoen P, Fleischer AB Jr. An evidence-based review of systemic treatments for itch. Eur J Pain 2016;20(1):24–31.
10. Grand'Maison S, Durand M, Mahone M. The effects of ursodeoxycholic acid treatment for intrahepatic cholestasis of pregnancy on maternal and fetal outcomes: a meta-analysis including non-randomized studies. J Obstet Gynaecol Can 2014;36:632–41.
11. Viegas LP, Ferreira MB, Kaplan AP. The maddening itch: an approach to chronic urticaria. J Investig Allergol Clin Immunol 2014;24:1–5.
12. Eichenfield LF, Tom WL, Berger TG, et al. Guidelines of care for the management of atopic dermatitis: section 2. Management and treatment of atopic dermatitis with topical therapies. J Am Acad Dermatol 2014;71:116–32.
13. Siemens W, Xander C, Meerpohl JJ, et al. Drug treatments for pruritus in adult palliative care. Dtsch Arztebl Int 2014;111:863–70.
14. Solak Y, Biyik Z, Atalay H, et al. Pregabalin versus gabapentin in the treatment of neuropathic pruritus in maintenance haemodialysis patients: a prospective, crossover study. Nephrology (Carlton) 2012;17:710–7.
15. Vila T, Gommer J, Scates AC. Role of gabapentin in the treatment of uremic pruritus. Ann Pharmacother 2008;42:1080–4.
16. Goutos I, Dziewulski P, Richardson PM. Pruritus in burns: review article. J Burn Care Res 2009;30:221–8.
17. Maciel AA, Cunha PR, Laraia IO, et al. Efficacy of gabapentin in the improvement of pruritus and quality of life of patients with notalgia paresthetica. An Bras Dermatol 2014;89:570–5.
18. Anand S. Gabapentin for pruritus in palliative care. Am J Hosp Palliat Care 2013;30:192–6.
19. Taranu T, Toader S, Esanu I, et al. Pruritus in the elderly. Pathophysiological, clinical, laboratory and therapeutic approach. Rev Med Chir Soc Med Nat Iasi 2014;118:33–8.
20. Xander C, Meerpohl JJ, Galandi D, et al. Pharmacological interventions for pruritus in adult palliative care patients. Cochrane Database Syst Rev 2013;(6):CD008320.
21. Yosipovitch G, Bernhard JD. Clinical practice. Chronic pruritus. N Engl J Med 2013;368:1625–34.

22. Yosipovitch G. Chronic pruritus: a paraneoplastic sign. Dermatol Ther 2010;23:590–6.

23. van Laarhoven AI, van der Sman-Mauriks IM, Donders AR, et al. Placebo effects on itch: a meta-analysis of clinical trials of patients with dermatological conditions. J Invest Dermatol 2015; 135:1234–43.

24. Schut C, Mollanazar NK, Kupfer J, et al. Psychological interventions in the treatment of chronic itch. Acta Derm Venereol 2016;96(2):157–61.

25. Hiramanek N. Itch: a symptom of occult disease. Aust Fam Physician 2004;33:495–9.

26. Berger TG, Shive M, Harper GM. Pruritus in the older patient: a clinical review. JAMA 2013;310:2443–50.

Contact Dermatitis
Practice Gaps and Challenges

Christen M. Mowad, MD

KEYWORDS

- Allergic contact dermatitis • Patch testing • Allergens • Screening allergen series

KEY POINTS

- Patch testing remains the criterion standard for diagnosing allergic contact dermatitis.
- Assessing patients for allergic contact dermatitis requires a detailed exposure history, expanded patch testing, 2 patch test readings, and thorough patient education.
- New chemicals are continually being added to the consumer's environment, and as such, physicians must be aware of the possibility of new allergens and test appropriately.
- Patch test screening series need to be updated to identify new allergens that are introduced into the consumer environment.

Patch testing has been the criterion standard for diagnosing allergic contact dermatitis (ACD) since the 1800s. The procedure itself has not changed significantly since it was first introduced. Allergens are placed on the upper back, left in place for 48 hours, removed, read, and reread 72 hours to 1 week later. Although the procedure itself might seem straightforward, patch testing performs best in the hands of those who are most familiar with the process and can maximize its usefulness. The actual application of the testing materials is only part of the procedure; allergen selection, interpretation, and the education of allergen avoidance are all significant components of the patch test procedure and are paramount to the successful management of the patient.

Practice gaps are unfortunately evident in the clinical practice of evaluating the patient suspected of ACD. Some of these practice gaps include the selection of allergens (which is in part dependent on allergen availability), how the testing procedure is performed, and what information is provided to the patient on completion of the test (**Box 1**). In addition, new chemicals are continuously being introduced into the marketplace and workplace, resulting in ongoing consumer exposure of potential new allergens presenting yet

> **Box 1**
> **Patch testing practice gaps**
>
> Allergen selection
>
> Patch test procedure
>
> Patient education
>
> Evolution of allergens

another set of challenges. A more recent issue has become the concern over potentially allergenic materials in metal implantable devices and how best to manage these situations. Appropriately evaluating these patients and providing useful information to the patient and referring surgeons is a daunting task.

The assessment of a patient suspected of ACD begins with a detailed and thorough patient history. The information obtained after this in-depth inquiry leads to allergen selection. Allergen selection presents a practice gap. Dermatologists across the country test to many different baseline screening series as well as to other expanded specialty series (**Box 2**). The decision of which screening series to use can be dependent on several factors, including allergen availability,

The author has nothing to disclose.
Department of Medicine, Division of Dermatology, Geisinger Medical Center, 115 Woodbine Lane, Danville, PA 17821, USA
E-mail address: cmowad@geisinger.edu

Dermatol Clin 34 (2016) 263–267
http://dx.doi.org/10.1016/j.det.2016.02.010

derm.theclinics.com

cost, and patient history. Studies have shown that the introduction of the US Food and Drug Administration (FDA) -approved preimpregnated allergen system, the thin-layer rapid use epicutaneous test (TRUE) test, has increased the use of patch testing among dermatologists, presumably due to increased ease of use.[1] The number of allergens in the FDA-approved testing series has increased over the years and now has 35 allergens and one control. Although a very good starting point, it can still miss up to 26.7% of allergens because of the limited number of allergens tested.[2] Even expanded series can miss relevant allergens, underscoring the need for a detailed and thorough history of exposures at home and in the workplace, including any potential consort exposures because this history may point to the need for a specialty tray of allergens (ie, dental tray, nail tray).[2] The continual introduction of new chemicals requires that the dermatologist remain vigilant and aware of new potential allergens in the patient's environment and test when appropriate. Not all dermatologists can maintain these expanded series. The practice gap of breadth and depth of allergen testing can be overcome through the understanding that negative testing to 35 allergens does not rule out ACD as a diagnosis and referral to centers with expertise in patch testing, and access to more allergens should be considered.

The influx of novel chemicals in the consumer environment results in the introduction of potential new allergens. This introduction of potential new allergens can lead to another potential practice gap. Not only must we test these new allergens in order to detect them, but also we must first be able to identify these allergens. One recent example was the successful identification of dimethyl fumarate as an allergen in multiple cases of "sofa dermatitis."[3] Several astute dermatologists were able to piece together the puzzle and identify the allergen as dimethyl fumarate, an antifungal, present in small sachets in the furniture.[3] The identification of this allergen closed the knowledge gap that existed and led to a change

in usage of this allergen, and as a result, this problem has largely been eliminated.

Another example of industry changes that led to the emergence of new allergens is seen in product preservation. In an ongoing effort to find the best preservative systems available (low cost, low toxicity, long shelf-life, and broad biocidal activity), industries introduce new chemicals into the marketplace. These new preservatives are potential new allergens. One can look to preservative usage databases to see this by the numbers. For example, formaldehyde and quaternium-15 have been widely used preservatives and over time have been found to be significant causes of ACD. As a result, these allergens have become less frequently used in personal care products, and new preservative systems have begun to replace them, demonstrated by corresponding increased usage numbers of these new chemicals.[4] Examples of some of these newer preservative allergens include methylisothiazolinone (MI), the allergen of the year 2013, and iodopropynyl butylcarbamate (IPBC). MI has traditionally been tested to as part of a mix, but in 2005 this chemical was approved as a stand-alone preservative. As a result, we are seeing more allergy to this chemical.[5] MI is not on the TRUE test and therefore can be missed if expanded testing is not performed to the chemical itself. IPBC was previously used as an industrial fungicide but was approved for use in cosmetics in the 1990s. This newer preservative system has been shown to cause ACD from usage in cosmetics.[6] These new chemicals have demonstrated their own ability to sensitize and cause ACD. Neither is on the FDA-approved screening series and would be missed unless they were tested for with expanded trays, highlighting the need for vigilance and awareness of the changing trends in allergen usage over time and the need to periodically update screening series so they remain current and useful in the ability to detect allergens and diagnose ACD.

Another example of industry change that effects consumer allergen exposure is evident in the fragrance arena. In 1977, fragrance mix I was introduced as a screening allergy to identify those allergic to fragrance.[7] This mix underwent its own evolution in order to be most helpful in detecting allergy to fragrance. However, over time, it has become less effective in detecting the newer fragrance chemicals that have entered the marketplace. As a result, fragrance mix II was developed in 2005 to screen for the newer fragrance chemicals.[8] Almost certainly, as more novel fragrances make their way into the marketplace, we will need to appropriately adjust and modify our screening allergens. Already newer fragrance allergens, such as linalool and limonene, are being reported.[9]

ACD to botanicals continues to be a challenge and a practice gap. Botanicals are increasingly being used in the personal care product market as consumers look for "natural" products. Screening for these chemicals is difficult because there are many botanicals and most are not adequately screened for by a single allergen. As a result, individual products and individual botanical allergens need to be used for patch testing in order to reliably detect allergy to a specific botanical. The patient exposure history becomes a critical part of the evaluation in order to identify any potential botanical allergens.

It is apparent that the introduction of new allergens in the marketplace will be a recurring event, and as a result, screening series must be adjusted and updated to reflect current usage patterns. The FDA-approved series has improved detection rates with the addition of key allergens. However, one must question how this screening series will hold up with its current composition as new allergens are introduced and seemingly problematic ones are phased out.

Education in the field has not changed dramatically. A recently conducted study did show that more faculty members designated as ACD experts are now members of the American Contact Dermatitis Society (ACDS), and ACD lectures are more routinely given in residency programs. Indications are also pointing to more expanded testing series being used by graduating residents, although this did not reach statistical significance.[10] The increase in ACD experts as members of the ACDS is likely due in large part to the robust database created by the society that is a valuable resource in patient education. The Contact Allergen Management System (CAMP) database is available on the ACDS Web site, www.contact-derm.org, and allows clinicians to enter a patient's known allergen(s) into a database that then screens products within the database, providing a list of products that are free of the patient's known allergens as well as any potential cross-reactors. This database streamlines the education process and makes compliance easier for the patient because it provides a "safe" list for them to shop with in addition to giving them the names of their identified allergens.

Although the patch test procedure itself has remained essentially the same over the years, in addition to allergen selection, there are several other practice gaps and challenges in the field. The patch test procedure involves application of the allergens to the upper back with occlusion for 48 hours during which time the allergens must be kept dry. At 48 hours, the patches should be removed in the office to insure that proper adherence of the patches occurred and to perform the first reading. The patient should then have a second patch test reading at 72 hours to 1 week later. Unfortunately, some gaps in care exist because this procedure is not always followed. Some patients are instructed on how to remove the patches at home, presumably to make fewer visits for the patient. However, this effort to increase patient convenience compromises the procedure. It does not allow for proper inspection of the patches to make sure that they remained in place and occluded, thereby insuring the integrity of the procedure. The second reading is also important because it helps discern between irritant and ACD and helps identify any late reactors. Unfortunately, this is another practice gap because second readings are not always conducted, most likely due to patient and/or provider convenience, and as many as 30% of allergens could be missed.[1] There are several potential late responders that will not be seen at the 48-hour reading, which means those not conducting a second patch test read may be missing these allergens and providing an incomplete assessment of the patient's allergy (**Box 3**). This gap in proper patch test procedure is likely due to convenience for patient and providers but needs to be adjusted in order for the patch test procedure to be properly performed and provide the most complete information.

The ongoing practice gap and knowledge gap of the reliability of patch testing performed while a patient is on immunosuppressive agents such as systemic steroids have been further complicated with the increased use of other immunosuppressive drugs and the new class of biologics. Although most physicians performing patch testing prefer a patient to be off prednisone for at least 1 week, many providers will test, when necessary, at the lowest dose possible, but preferably less than 10 mg per day.[11-13] The use of other immunosuppressive agents, such as mycophenolate mofetil, methotrexate, azathioprine, cyclosporine, and tumor necrosis factor-α inhibitors,

Box 3
Some allergens with possible delayed reactions
Bacitracin
Disperse blue dyes
Cocamidopropyl betaine
Corticosteroids
P-Phenylenediamine

does not appear to be an absolute contraindication to patch testing.[13-15] Testing at the lowest possible dose is recommended and 2+ and 3+ reactions are most reliable. When patch testing patients on these medications, one must consider the possibility of suppressed, or weak but relevant reactions.

Once allergens are identified, education is key to the management of the patient. Simply providing the names of the allergens to a patient compromises the usefulness of the patch test procedure. Patient education varies widely and is another practice gap issue. Dermatologists must educate and explain the allergens to the patient including any synonyms, where the allergen is likely to be found as well as possible cross-reacting chemicals that may need to be avoided. Providing a narrative sheet with this information is very helpful. Narrative sheets can be found in English and Spanish on the ACDS Web site. Another extremely valuable tool is the previously mentioned CAMP database available to members on the same Web site. This database provides patients with a list of "safe" products free of their known allergens and any cross-reactors. This database makes it much easier for patients to comply with avoidance. Follow-up visits to reinforce allergen avoidance and review progress are essential in the management of these patients.

A more recent and increasingly common question is the application and usefulness of patch testing in the evaluation and management of patients with metal devices. Dermatologists are increasingly being asked to patch test patients before the implantation of a metal device. This request sometimes comes from the concerned patient but is now more frequently coming from a referring surgeon who requires the testing before surgery. The controversy over patch testing and metal devices and how best to assist these patients and their surgeons remains a topic of debate. This topic of debate is seen in cardiology, in dental practices, and in thoracic surgery but is most apparent in orthopedics. With the rising number of joints being replaced in this country each year, it is perhaps not surprising that metal allergy has become a hot issue. The question of how patch testing in its current form can best assist these patients remains to be determined. Other tests, such as the lymphocyte transformation assay, may be useful to help answer these questions; however, these studies are costly, not widely available, and often not covered by insurance.

Knowing how best to manage these patients, and when to use patch testing in this situation, remains a practice gap without significant evidence-based data to guide clinicians. The dermatologist must set realistic expectations and educate the surgeon and the patient on the limitations of this procedure. Patch testing is a cutaneous test that does not re-create the environment of the metal device, may not provide information relative to the implanted device, and is therefore limited in the information it can provide. It is also not predictive of future allergy and only provides information about the patient's current state of sensitivity.

The question of preimplant testing for those with a history of metal allergy appears the most straightforward but still raises several concerns and questions. If a patient has a history of metal allergy, testing them to metals and reporting any allergens to the surgeon in order for these allergens to be avoided if possible seems reasonable. There are, however, reports of nickel-allergic patients with implants that contain nickel that are problem free.[16] One must ask if a history of metal allergy or positive preimplantation testing is directing the surgeon to choose more expensive devices, or less durable device, even though no clear correlation between allergy and complication exists; this should be a concern given the significant number of joints replaced yearly and the resultant cost to society. Prospective studies evaluating the outcomes of those individuals with and without preimplant testing, impact of joint selection, and surgical outcomes are needed to help guide clinicians but are not yet available.[17-20]

Postimplant testing is even more complicated. Patients who are suffering from joint failure, joint pain or loosening, dermatitis over the implant, or more diffuse dermatitis are sometimes referred for patch testing to assess for possible ACD to the metal device. If patch testing detects a metal allergen, it is not possible to determine if the metal allergy caused the problem, or if the problem, such as loosening of a joint, resulted in sensitization. When an allergy is found in a patient with a static metal device, such as a plate, cause and effect seems more apparent, and removal of the metal can result in resolution.[20] It is much more difficult to determine causation in the other situations. Decisions to remove or replace metal devices must be made with the surgeon and patient taking into consideration all the risks of another procedure with no guarantee of improvement. Clearly more evidence-based data are needed, and in the meantime, consensus expert opinion recommendations are being developed to help guide clinicians.

Patch testing has been an in-office procedure since the 1800s, and although the actual procedure has not changed considerably during that time, several challenges remain. Throughout the environment, we are exposed to hundreds of

Table 1
Patch testing best practices

Best Practice	Best Practice Strategies	Barriers to Best Practice
Expanded screening series	Obtain expanded series Referral centers	Cost, availability of allergens
Two patch test reads	Schedule 2 patch test reads	Time/convenience
Patch test off immunosuppressives	Patch test off immunosuppressives	Inability to wean off medicines

allergens daily, and new allergens will continually be introduced into our personal care products and our workplace. Our ability to detect relevant allergens necessitates that we routinely update and change our screening series in order to keep current with new allergens. Furthermore, as medicine continues to make advances, our bodies will be exposed to new and different chemicals and devices. We need to better identify the role of patch testing in these settings in order to best serve the needs of our patients (**Table 1**).

REFERENCES

1. Warshaw EM, Moore JB, Nelson D. Prevalence of patch testing and methodology of dermatologists in the US: results of a cross- sectional survey. Am J Contact Dermat 2002;13(2):53–8.
2. Warshaw EM, Belsito DV, Taylor JS, et al. North American contact dermatitis group patch test results: 2009-2010. Dermatitis 2013;24(2):50–9.
3. Bruze M, Zimerson E. Dimethyl fumarate. Dermatitis 2011;22(1):3–7.
4. Steinberg DC. 2010 frequency of preservative use. Cosmet Toiletries 2010;125(11):46–51.
5. Castanedo-Tardana MP, Zug KA. Methylisothiazolinone. Dermatitis 2013;24(1):2–6.
6. Pazzaglia M, Tosti A. Allergic contact dermatitis from 3-iodo-2-propynyl-butylcarbamate in a cosmetic cream. Contact Dermatitis 1999;41(5):290.
7. Larsen WG. Perfume dermatitis. J Am Acad Dermatol 1985;12(10):1–9.
8. Heisterberg MV, Andersen KE, Avnstorp C, et al. Fragrance mix II as a marker of identifying fragrance allergy. Contact Dermatitis 2010;63:270–6.
9. Cheng J, Zug KA. Fragrance allergic contact dermatitis. Dermatitis 2014;25(5):232–45.
10. Nelson J, Mowad C, Sun H. Allergic contact dermatitis and patch-testing education in US dermatology residences in 2010. Dermatitis 2012;23(2):56–60.
11. Feuerman E, Levy A. A study of the effect of prednisone and an antihistamine on patch test reactions. Br J Dermatol 1972;86(1):68–71.
12. Anveden I, Lindberg M, Andersen KE, et al. Oral prednisone suppresses allergic but not irritant patch test reactions in individuals hypersensitive to nickel. Contact Dermatitis 2004; 50(5):298–303.
13. Fowler JF, Maibach HI, Zirwas M, et al. Effects of immunomodulatory agents on patch testing: expert opinion 2012. Dermatitis 2012; 23(6):301–2.
14. Rosmarin D, Gottlieb AB, Asarch A, et al. Patch-testing while on systemic immunosuppressants. Dermatitis 2009;20(5):265–70.
15. Wee JS, White JML, McFadden JP, et al. Patch testing in patients treated with systemic immunosuppression and cytokine inhibitors. Contact Dermatitis 2010;62(3):165–9.
16. Carlsson A, Moller A. Implantation of orthopedic devices in patients with metal allergy. Acta Derm Venereol 1989;69:62–6.
17. Schalock PC. Pragmatism and the evaluation of metal hypersensitivity reactions. Dermatitis 2013; 24:104–5.
18. Thyssen JP, Menne T, Schalock PC, et al. Pragmatic approach to the clinical work-up of patients with putative allergic disease to metallic orthopedic implants before and after surgery. Br J Dermatol 2011;164:473–8.
19. Crawford GH. The role of patch testing in the evaluation of orthopedic implant-related adverse effects: current evidence does not support broad use. Dermatitis 2013;24(3):99–111.
20. Atanaskova Mesinkovska N, Tellez A, Molina L, et al. The effect of patch testing on surgical practices and outcomes in orthopedic patients with metal implants. Arch Dermatol 2012;148(6):687–93.

Clinical and Educational Gaps in Diagnosis of Nail Disorders

Anna Q. Hare, MD[a], Phoebe Rich, MD[b,c],*

KEYWORDS

- Nail surgery • Nail biopsy • Nail disorders • Nail dystrophy

KEY POINTS

- Improving resident exposure to diverse nail disease processes and diagnostic procedures will initially require creativity to increase experience with limited exposure.
- The main hurdle to overcome in increasing resident exposure to nail pathology/procedure is simply the current low volume seen in some residencies.
- Although the capacity and desire of residencies to handle nail procedures increases over time, other modes of experience may aid in building confidence among residents.

PRACTICE AND EDUCATIONAL GAPS IN DISORDERS OF THE NAILS IN DERMATOLOGY

Introduction

Dermatologists are experts in the care of skin, hair and nails, yet many dermatologists find nails challenging and even frustrating. Nail disorders are sometimes considered trivial, and nail procedures can be labor intensive and poorly reimbursed compared with many other skin procedures. Well-recognized disease processes on the skin may seem clinically different when involving the nail unit; nail biopsies are more involved and take longer than skin biopsies, and the slow growth of nails results in a longer wait to evaluate the treatment effect than on the skin. Furthermore, our collective knowledge of the basic science of structure, function, and pathophysiology of the nail unit lags behind that of the hair follicle, adnexal structures, and skin. Research in nails is a growing field with new interest in nail matrix stem cell potential. However, clinical and surgical nail experience in resident education continues to lag,

resulting in limited nail differential diagnoses in clinical practice, potential for missed or misdiagnosed nail disease, and lack of confidence in performing nail biopsies.

PRACTICE GAPS IN CLINICAL DERMATOLOGY: DIAGNOSIS OF NAIL PATHOLOGY

Best Practice

1. Dermatologists are able to diagnose the full spectrum of nail diseases, including infectious, neoplastic, congenital, inflammatory, traumatic, and those associated with systemic disease in a timely manner.
2. Dermatologists are confident in performing diagnostic nail surgical procedures; they know when, where, why, and how to perform a nail biopsy.

Current Clinical Practice

Current clinical practice gaps in diagnosing nail problems stem from a lack of appreciation of the

Conflict of Interest Statement: No conflicts of interest.
[a] Department of Dermatology, Oregon Health and Science University, Mail Code CH16D, 3303 Southwest Bond Avenue, Portland, OR 97239, USA; [b] Department of Dermatology, Oregon Health and Science University, 3181 SW Sam Jackson Park Rd, Portland, OR 97239, USA; [c] Oregon Dermatology Research Center, 2565 Northwest Lovejoy Street, Portland, OR 97210, USA
* Corresponding author.
E-mail addresses: phoeberich@aol.com; rich@ohsu.edu

Dermatol Clin 34 (2016) 269–273
http://dx.doi.org/10.1016/j.det.2016.02.002
0733-8635/16/$ – see front matter © 2016 Elsevier Inc. All rights reserved.

broad range of nail diagnoses as well as a lack of knowledge of clinical and procedural techniques for diagnosis of nail disease processes, leading to discomfort surrounding diagnosis and management of complex nail disorders. Although 50% of nail conditions seen in a general medical dermatology office are fungal, the other 50% are something other than fungal, including neoplastic, inflammatory, congenital, traumatic, or related to systemic disease.[1] Because some of these nonfungal conditions resemble onychomycosis clinically, they may be consequently initially misdiagnosed and even treated, exposing patients to unnecessary systemic antifungal drugs and possibly delaying important diagnosis. Further delay ensues when patients are referred outside our specialty for fingernail or toenail procedures, which are not infrequent occurrences in busy clinics when dermatologists are either not interested or not confident in treating nail disorders and performing nail biopsies.

The knowledge and attitude gap: delay in diagnosis of nail conditions

Lack of appreciation of the number and wide variety of nail disorders leads to an early limited differential and sometimes dismissal, when instead the initial differential should be broad and properly explored. This clinical practice gap spans both attitude toward and knowledge of nail physiology and the breadth of nail disease processes. For example, there is overall a lack of knowledge of the proper differential diagnosis and workup of nail dyschromia. Longitudinal melanonychia and longitudinal erythronychia can be the result of a benign or malignant process. Subungual melanomas and squamous cell carcinoma of the nail unit may present subtly with only

onycholysis or longitudinal dyschromia and, consequently, are often unrecognized early (**Figs. 1** and **2**). Malignant tumors of the nail, although uncommon, are often advanced when diagnosed because the early signs were not recognized and the nail was not biopsied in a timely manner.[2–4] The consideration, workup, and treatment of these less-common but high-stakes conditions are crucial elements of good patient care in dermatology.

Narrowing the Gap

Current gaps in clinical nail diseaes diagnosis can be significantly narrowed with a 2-pronged approach to address both knowledge and attitude. Clinical diagnosis, including maintaining a broad early differential and appropriately considering harmful disease processes would improve with a standardized approach to nail disease diagnosis. Algorithms that use clinical signs and symptoms of an abnormal nail to arrive at the correct diagnosis for a wide range of nail disorders could significantly improve the aforementioned practice gaps. An algorithmic approach to nail diagnosis should strictly adhere to the core principles of confirming the presence of organisms before diagnosing onychomycosis and encourage diligent consideration of other possible diagnoses until the organism is definitively noted. Algorithms that use examination and history of nail disease signs and symptoms to assist with diagnosis and clinical decision-making are currently lacking. Gaps in attitude regarding the importance of nail conditions could be addressed by increased didactic nail sessions at the American Academy of Dermatology and other regional meetings as well as further assessment of nail burden of disease, using

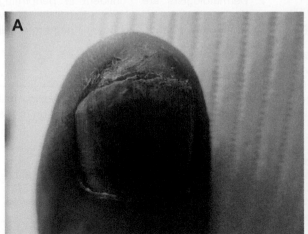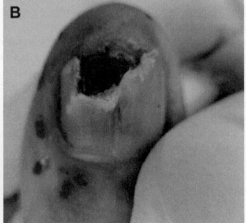

Fig. 1. Amelanotic melanoma of the nail bed presenting as onycholysis and treated as an infection for 2 years before nail biopsy.

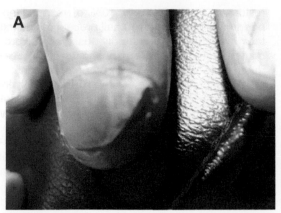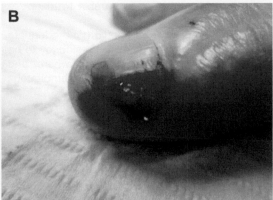

Fig. 2. (*A, B*) Invasive squamous cell carcinoma of nail bed requiring amputation. Lesion was previously treated as a pyogenic granuloma.

electronic medical record data, in the clinic patient population. This increased focus and evaluation would highlight the important place of nail disease diagnosis in best practice in clinical dermatology.

The skill and attitude gap: confidence in knowing when, where, and how to perform diagnostic and therapeutic nail surgical procedures

Monodactylous nail disorders must be considered potentially neoplastic. Confidence, knowledge, and interest regarding nail biopsy once neoplasm is suspected is the next step in the timely diagnosis of nail pathologic process (see **Figs. 1** and **2**). This gap encompasses skill (in knowing when and how to biopsy) and attitude (the recognition that this is an important aspect of clinical dermatology practice). Many neoplastic nail disorders are referred out to hand surgeons and podiatrists because of the lack of interest or confidence in performing nail biopsies in the clinic, resulting in a delay in diagnosis.[5] Current skill and attitude gaps regarding nail diagnostic procedures stems partly from our limited knowledge of nail physiology. A firm understanding of the anatomy of the nail unit and how location of the pathologic process in the nail unit drives characteristic clinical features of a nail problem is underappreciated. Knowledge of nail physiology assists with knowing when and where to biopsy a dystrophic nail by understanding that abnormalities in certain areas of the nail unit yields characteristic clinical features. For example, pitting and leukonychia are caused by identical disease process in the proximal and distal nail matrix, respectively. Unfortunately, many nails are biopsied in the wrong location in the nail unit and abnormality entirely miss important evidence of the disease process. Even more than in the skin, biopsy of the correct part of a

nail lesion is crucial for correct diagnosis.[6,7] With current basic science of the nail lagging behind that of other adnexal structures, confidence in our knowledge of causative factors in nail disease naturally wavers. Understanding nail growth kinetics and the properties and interactions between the nail matrix and the nail bed are crucial for a logical diagnosis.

Narrowing the Gap

Improving knowledge of nail physiology is the first step in increasing our confidence in the diagnosis of diseases of the nail unit pathologic processes, yet currently there is little focus on nail physiology in either basic science or resident education. Steps to narrow this knowledge gap and, thus, increase confidence in clinic-performed diagnostic procedures can be taken in both the basic science realm and in education. Exploration of the potential of nail matrix stem cells both increases our knowledge of pathologic nail processes as well as brings a greater awareness and appreciation to the basic anatomy and physiology of the nail. Increased emphasis in resident education on nail procedures will be crucial for narrowing this procedural gap over time (see later discussion). Increased didactic sessions at the medical meetings, cadaver dissection of digits, and live nail surgery demonstrations can start to narrow this gap in current practice, bringing confidence to clinical diagnosis and diagnostic procedures.

EDUCATIONAL GAP (IN DERMATOLOGY RESIDENCY EDUCATION)
Best Practice

1. Dermatology residents should have sufficient experience with a wide variety of nail conditions

during their residency to be able to diagnose and treat any nail condition.

2. Dermatology residents should have adequate nail surgery experience during residency to be comfortable knowing when, why, where, and how to perform a nail biopsy on an ambiguous nail dystrophy.

Current Practice: Lack of Resident Exposure to Nail Disease Diagnosis and Diagnostic Procedures

Many dermatologists do not have the training and experience to perform nail procedures confidently. This training and experience should begin in residency. Currently there is a wide spectrum of exposure to nail disease and diagnosis in residency, but overall exposure remains inadequate to build confidence surrounding nails in clinical practice. Residents are often not taught how to work up a nail dystrophy to arrive at a differential diagnosis based on history and clinical nail morphology. Further, they are often not taught to use clinical morphology to determine the location and method of biopsy. Finally, lack of exposure to adequate nail procedures during residency precludes confidence in performing nail procedures.

Assessing the Gap

Some residents receive insufficient hands-on experience performing nail procedures, resulting in a practice-based learning gap. Few training programs have a nail expert on the faculty, and often there is little identification of the nail as a specialized area of diagnosis and procedure. Workup and diagnosis of nail disease are often taught in a piecemeal fashion within other categories of dermatology with little focus on using knowledge of nail physiology to aid in diagnosis. Residents may have less exposure to nail disease when cases are referred to community physicians with a nail specialty or to fields outside of dermatology, such as hand surgeons or podiatrists.[5] For a variety of reasons, resident exposure to nail disease workup and biopsy is lacking, limiting practice-based learning in residency.

As the number of procedures performed by dermatologists has increased, over the past 15 years there has been an increase in requirements to ensure adequate procedural training during residency. Despite the increased focus on procedural dermatology, there remains a dearth of nail surgery experience in residency education. Based on a survey in 2009 of 240 third-year residents representing 89% of all US dermatology residency programs, only 10% of respondents performed greater than 10 nail procedures during their residency, 25% had only observed nail procedures, and 4% were exposed to nail procedures only via lecture. Thirty-three percent of residents performed fewer than 5 nerve blocks of any type. Thirty percent rated themselves not competent to perform nail surgery (only surgery with flaps and grafts yielded lower confidence). Yet when surveyed, greater than 75% of respondents in a survey of residents in 2004 rated nail biopsy as an essential procedure to learn in residency.[8]

Narrowing the Gap

Improving resident exposure to diverse nail diseaes processes and diagnostic procedures will initially require creativity to increase experience with limited exposure. The main hurdle to overcome in increasing resident exposure to nail disease and diagnostic procedures is simply the current low volume seen in some residencies. In time it will be important to reverse this trend by starting to do more nail procedures. Although the capacity and desire of residencies to handle nail procedures increases over time, other modes of experience may aid in building confidence among residents. Some residency programs are now using cadaver nails or artificial nail models to teach residents nail surgery techniques.[9,10] Other programs that do not have a nail specialist on faculty have affiliated with community dermatologists to increase resident exposure.

REFERENCES

1. Lipner SR, Scher RK. Onychomycosis - a small step for quality of care. Current Medical Research and Opinion 2016;1–3.

2. Di Chiacchio N, Hirata SH, Enokihara MY, et al. Dermatologists' accuracy in early diagnosis of melanoma of the nail matrix. Arch Dermatol 2010;146(4): 382–7.

3. Soon SL, Solomon AR Jr, Papadopoulos D, et al. Acral lentiginous melanoma mimicking benign disease: the Emory experience. J Am Acad Dermatol 2003;48(2):183–8.

4. Winslet M, Tejan J. Subungual amelanotic melanoma: a diagnostic pitfall. Postgrad Med J 1990;66(773): 200–2.

5. Velez NF, Jellinek NJ. Nailing it: promoting nail procedural training in residency and beyond. Dermatol Surg 2015;41(3):424–6.

6. de Berker DA, Dahl MG, Comaish JS, et al. Nail surgery: an assessment of indications and outcome. Acta Derm Venereol 1996;76(6):484–7.

7. Rich P. Nail biopsy: indications and methods. Dermatol Surg 2001;27(3):229–34.

8. Lee EH, Nehal KS, Dusza SW, et al. Procedural dermatology training during dermatology residency: a survey of third-year dermatology residents. J Am Acad Dermatol 2011;64(3):475–83, 83.e1–5.

9. Pate DA, Shimizu I. Not just nail polish: inexpensive reusable model for practicing nail procedures. Dermatol Surg 2015;41(3):423–4.

10. Clark M, YS, Kundu R. Nail surgery techniques: a single center survey on the effect of a cadaveric hand practicum in dermatology resident education. Dermatologic Surgery, in press.

Practice and Educational Gaps in Dermatology
Disorders of the Hair

Maria L. Colavincenzo, MD

KEYWORDS

- Hair patients • Practice gaps • Dermoscopy of the scalp and hair

KEY POINTS

- Several clinical practice gaps exist in the care of hair patients.
- Attitude gaps include a relative lack of dermatologists interested in caring for patients with hair complaints, a potential underestimation of the effect of hair disorders on the quality of patients' lives, and potential failure to recognize the presentation of body dysmorphic disorder among patients with hair complaints.
- Knowledge gaps regarding the prevalence and presentation of hair loss disorders, particularly cicatricial alopecias such as frontal fibrosing alopecia and central centrifugal cicatricial alopecia, may lead to a delay in diagnosis and treatment of hair patients.
- Skill gaps in physical examination, particularly lack of comfort with dermoscopy of the scalp and hair, may affect the care of hair patients.
- Many practice gaps exist regarding uncertainty as to the ideal management of both nonscarring and particularly scarring alopecias.

PRACTICE GAP
Attitude Gaps

Although general dermatologists are trained as experts in disorders of the hair, skin, and nails, there are unique challenges in caring for hair patients. One of the most significant gaps in dermatologists' care for patients with hair disorders is a fundamental one: a relative lack of dermatologists interested in caring for patients with hair complaints, which may limit patient access to care. Potential barriers to caring for hair patients are many and may include provider perception of visits for hair concerns as time-consuming, with strong emotional undertones, often without simple or rapid treatment options for the patients' conditions. These challenges may seem even more difficult in the current and evolving health care environment, where clinical efficiency and quantifiable positive outcomes may be stressed, steering some dermatologists away from the care of patients with hair disorders altogether, and others toward boutique practices out of reach financially for many patients, potentially limiting the availability of expert care.

An era has been entered into that promises continued strides in the basic science understanding and clinical therapeutic developments toward treating the range of hair disorders, with remarkable recent progress regarding some of the most common hair disorders, including appreciating the role of the janus kinase pathway in alopecia areata,[1,2] prostaglandins in androgenetic alopecia,[3,4] and a possible therapeutic role for platelet-rich plasma,[5,6] to give but a few examples. Increasing awareness of and enthusiasm regarding these advancements going forward

The author has no commercial/financial conflicts of interest nor funding sources to disclose.
Department of Dermatology, Northwestern University Feinberg School of Medicine, 676 North St Clair Street, Suite 1600, Chicago, IL 60611, USA
E-mail address: mcolavi1@nm.org

Dermatol Clin 34 (2016) 275–279
http://dx.doi.org/10.1016/j.det.2016.02.003

may serve to combat at least some of the barriers affecting providers' attitudes toward caring for hair patients in the future. Practical solutions to facilitate the care of hair patients include spreading complaints over multiple visits to enable dedicating adequate time to address patients' concerns.

Two other significant attitude gaps are notable in the care of hair patients. The first is a potential underestimation of the effect of hair disorders of the quality of patients' lives. There is the concept of "the difficult hair loss patient,"[7] yet there may be among providers a tendency to perceive hair loss as a relatively trivial problem, a failure to grasp the dramatic consequences that hair loss can have on patients' lives. Moreover, the author found that providers' perceived severity of a patient's hair loss does not correlate with the impact on quality of life, and even objectively mild alopecia may be a significant detriment to quality of life.[8] In a growing body of literature, many conditions commonly managed by dermatologists, quintessentially psoriasis and atopic dermatitis, have been shown to have great effects on quality of life[9,10]; thus, dermatologists are increasingly familiar with the concept of assessing quality of life in the management of cutaneous disorders. Application of the same sensitivity in assessing alopecia patients, whether through careful history taking or dedicated screening surveys, may lead to better overall care of these patients.

A second gap in the care of hair patients might also be addressed with increased screening as to emotional and psychological health states: the potential failure to recognize the presentation of body dysmorphic disorder (BDD) among patients with hair complaints. BDD is a psychiatric condition with significant impact on patients' health and survival, including a high prevalence of suicidality among patients.[11] Although patients with BDD are likely overrepresented in dermatology clinics in general because of the visible nature of the complaints in this field,[12,13] recent reports suggest that the prevalence of BDD among patients with hair complaints is significantly higher than among general dermatology patients.[14] Screening for BDD among hair patients may serve to identify those at increased risk and who may benefit most from treatment of their underlying psychiatric condition, above and beyond treatments directed at their perceived hair disorders. Barriers to inquiring as to the emotional and psychiatric state of hair patients relate primarily to the perception that significant additional time would be needed in an already time-consuming visit. However, brief screening instruments have been validated in dermatology patients,[15] and patients with BDD,

in the long run, will not be managed effectively or efficiently without addressing the underlying mental health state.

Knowledge Gaps

Knowledge gaps may affect the care of patients with both scarring and nonscarring alopecias, delaying accurate diagnosis and appropriate treatment. In the case of scarring alopecias, particularly frontal fibrosing alopecia (FFA) and central centrifugal cicatricial alopecia (CCCA), patients often suffer from a delay in diagnosis. With any scarring process, a delay in diagnosis is particularly problematic because it can mean a missed opportunity to prevent progressive and often permanent alopecia.

FFA, first described in 1994 as a unique subtype of lichen planopilaris primarily affecting postmenopausal Caucasian women,[16] has undergone a dramatic increase in incidence in recent years.[17,18] The factors underlying this remarkable change remain largely unknown. Furthermore, with the increase of FFA, the condition is no longer restricted to postmenopausal Caucasian women, but has now been reported in women of various skin types and ethnic backgrounds, many premenopausal, and there are increasing reports of FFA in male patients (Figs. 1–3).

General dermatologists should be aware of this recent dynamic and be on the lookout for this once rare but increasingly prevalent condition, which may present initially with somewhat subtle clinical findings. Potentially confounding the clinical diagnosis of FFA, despite its designation as a subtype of lichen planopilaris, often the expected symptoms and signs of inflammation (pain or pruritus, perifollicular papules, erythema, or scale) may be minimal. Biopsies from seemingly inactive FFA often reveal an active underlying process, and patients will continue to lose hair.

Especially when the signs of inflammation are subtle, FFA may be misdiagnosed, often as

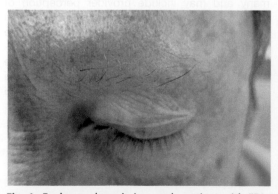

Fig. 1. Eyebrow alopecia in a male patient with FFA.

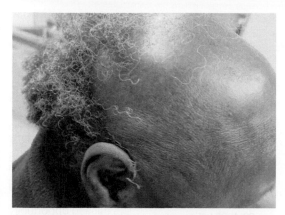

Fig. 2. Severe scarring alopecia in an African American woman with FFA.

androgenetic alopecia or alopecia areata. Close inspection of the eyebrows and frontal hairline for subtle clues may aid in detecting FFA in an earlier state. In the absence of obvious inflammatory papules, these may include frontal hairline alopecia in association with eyebrow alopecia, and a rather pathognomonic "lonely hair sign" of isolated remaining terminal hairs at the scarred hairline.[19] Given the expectation of hairline recession related to androgenetic alopecia in male patients, loss of beard, sideburn, or eyebrow hair is the more likely presenting complaint in this group (and can be misdiagnosed as alopecia areata). Finally, associated skin-colored facial papules have been described and represent FFA affecting the facial hair follicles,[20] which may be another clue. A high level of suspicion and low threshold to biopsy when the diagnosis of FFA is being considered may prevent delayed diagnosis.

CCCA is another cicatricial alopecia wherein knowledge gaps may delay diagnosis and appropriate treatment. CCCA is a common cause of hair loss among African American women,

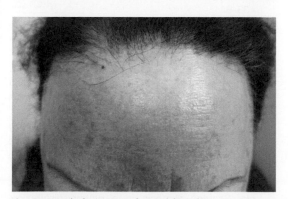

Fig. 3. Lonely hair sign, frontal hair line recession in an Asian American woman with FFA.

typically starting in the crown or central scalp.[21,22] The exact causes and pathological mechanisms remain unclear, with a possible but uncertain role of hair practices in disease progression. Patients may or may not have symptoms of scalp tenderness, pruritus, or sensitivity preceding or accompanying clinically obvious alopecia. Especially in cases of asymptomatic alopecia, this diagnosis may not be considered early on. Because the common distribution of CCCA over the crown overlaps with distribution of female pattern hair loss, early CCCA may be misdiagnosed as female pattern/androgenetic alopecia and not recognized until there has been significant progression of irreversible scarring. Clues to CCCA may include a subtle shininess or smooth quality to the alopecic scalp (from scarring over of follicular ostia), and any signs of inflammation, such as erythema, perifollicular hyperpigmentation, scale, or edema. More recently, focal hair breakage on the crown has been described as a potential early sign of CCCA.[23]

Skill Gap

Another potential gap affecting the care of hair patients may relate to level of comfort with dermoscopic evaluation of the scalp and hair (trichoscopy). In recent years, appreciation of the potential role of dermoscopy in the evaluation of dermatologic conditions has extended far beyond neoplastic conditions to include a wide range of inflammatory and noninflammatory processes, among them the hair disorders. From hair shaft miniaturization to "yellow dots" to vascular patterns, a wealth of recent literature has elucidated a whole new realm of potentially useful examination findings.[24,25] Because dermoscopy is an acquired skill with a learning curve, the ability to recognize and incorporate these findings into a routine scalp assessment remains an area where many dermatologists may not yet feel confident. With time, practice, and clarification of these patterns via further study, it is likely that the role of trichoscopy in the care of hair patients will continue to blossom in the future.

Specific Practice Gaps: Treatment

The treatment of hair disorders is fraught with many practice gaps regarding uncertainty as to the ideal management of both nonscarring and particularly scarring alopecias. Nearly every common hair disorder has an associated practice gap related to an overall paucity of evidence-based treatment options. Common clinical scenarios leave many currently unanswered questions: When topical minoxidil and oral antiandrogens are not effective in curtailing androgenetic alopecia, the most common hair disorder affecting millions of men and women, what other options do we have? What should we do when intralesional steroid injections are not effective in alopecia areata, and how should we treat extensive cases, such as alopecia totalis and alopecia universalis? What is the proper algorithm for treatment of CCCA, FFA? Can anything help seemingly "burned out scarring alopecia," and is there a role for hair transplant or stem cell therapy in the future?

These questions are just some of the myriad of remaining questions facing dermatologists who manage hair disorders, and these incompletely answered questions about treatment remain perhaps the most significant gap in clinical practice. If the current pace of investigation and discovery continues, there is optimism that today's research will ultimately inform these questions in the not-so-distant future, with the potential to bridge some of the many gaps in the clinical care for hair patients.

EDUCATION GAP (IN DERMATOLOGY RESIDENT EDUCATION)

Ideally, residents would, over the course of their residency, have a broad exposure to the range of hair disorders and become comfortable and proficient in the diagnosis, workup, and management of these conditions. In reality, residents may complete residency without gaining this experience and confidence, largely related to the practice gaps identified above, which affect dermatologists in both private and academic settings. When dermatology faculty have diminished interest in treating hair patients and failure to appreciate the impact of these conditions on patients' lives and psychiatric well-being, these attitudes are easily communicated to and assimilated by residents. Similarly, if dermatology faculty are not themselves confident in their ability to evaluate patients with hair disorders, and with the evolving nuances of diagnosis and treatment, then residents will not acquire this knowledge and skill. Thus, the educational gaps with regard to disorders of the hair very closely mirror the gaps in best clinical practice, and the measures to overcome them are largely the same. Our residents can be encouraged to see hair patients, inquire about their lives, pick up their dermatoscopes to look for subtle diagnostic clues, and stay abreast of and engage in the process of inquiry and research, in hopes of illuminating some of the many remaining gaps in the care of hair patients in the future.

REFERENCES

1. Jabbari A, Dai Z, Xing L, et al. Reversal of alopecia areata following treatment with the JAK1/2 inhibitor baricitinib. EBioMedicine 2015;2(4):351–5.
2. Xing L, Dai Z, Jabbari A, et al. Alopecia areata is driven by cytotoxic T lymphocytes and is reversed by JAK inhibition. Nat Med 2014;20(9):1043–9.
3. Garza LA, Liu Y, Yang Z, et al. Prostaglandin D2 inhibits hair growth and is elevated in bald scalp of men with androgenetic alopecia. Sci Transl Med 2012;4(126):126ra134.
4. Nieves A, Garza LA. Does prostaglandin D2 hold the cure to male pattern baldness? Exp Dermatol 2014; 23(4):224–7.
5. Maria-Angeliki G, Alexandros-Efstratios K, Dimitris R, et al. Platelet-rich plasma as a potential treatment for noncicatricial alopecias. Int J Trichology 2015;7(2): 54–63.
6. Schiavone G, Raskovic D, Greco J, et al. Platelet-rich plasma for androgenetic alopecia: a pilot study. Dermatol Surg 2014;40(9):1010–9.
7. Trueb RM. The difficult hair loss patient: a particular challenge. Int J Trichology 2013;5(3):110–4.
8. Reid EE, Haley AC, Borovicka JH, et al. Clinical severity does not reliably predict quality of life in women with alopecia areata, telogen effluvium, or androgenic alopecia. J Am Acad Dermatol 2012; 66(3):e97–102.
9. Ben-Gashir MA, Seed PT, Hay RJ. Quality of life and disease severity are correlated in children with atopic dermatitis. Br J Dermatol 2004;150(2): 284–90.
10. Garshick MK, Kimball AB. Psoriasis and the life cycle of persistent life effects. Dermatol Clin 2015; 33(1):25–39.
11. Cotterill JA, Cunliffe WJ. Suicide in dermatological patients. Br J Dermatol 1997;137(2):246–50.
12. Dogruk Kacar S, Ozuguz P, Bagcioglu E, et al. The frequency of body dysmorphic disorder in dermatology and cosmetic dermatology clinics: a study from Turkey. Clin Exp Dermatol 2014;39(4): 433–8.
13. Phillips KA, Dufresne RG. Body dysmorphic disorder. A guide for dermatologists and cosmetic surgeons. Am J Clin Dermatol 2000;1(4):235–43.
14. Dogruk Kacar S, Ozuguz P, Bagcioglu E, et al. Frequency of body dysmorphic disorder among patients with complaints of hair loss. Int J Dermatol 2016;55(4):425–9.
15. Picavet V, Gabriels L, Jorissen M, et al. Screening tools for body dysmorphic disorder in a cosmetic surgery setting. Laryngoscope 2011;121(12): 2535–41.
16. Kossard S. Postmenopausal frontal fibrosing alopecia. Scarring alopecia in a pattern distribution. Arch Dermatol 1994;130(6):770–4.

17. MacDonald A, Clark C, Holmes S. Frontal fibrosing alopecia: a review of 60 cases. J Am Acad Dermatol 2012;67(5):955–61.

18. Vano-Galvan S, Molina-Ruiz AM, Serrano-Falcon C, et al. Frontal fibrosing alopecia: a multicenter review of 355 patients. J Am Acad Dermatol 2014;70(4): 670–8.

19. Fernandez-Crehuet P, Rodrigues-Barata AR, Vano-Galvan S, et al. Trichoscopic features of frontal fibrosing alopecia: results in 249 patients. J Am Acad Dermatol 2015;72(2):357–9.

20. Donati A, Molina L, Doche I, et al. Facial papules in frontal fibrosing alopecia: evidence of vellus follicle involvement. Arch Dermatol 2011;147(12):1424–7.

21. Ogunleye TA, McMichael A, Olsen EA. Central centrifugal cicatricial alopecia: what has been achieved, current clues for future research. Dermatol Clin 2014;32(2):173–81.

22. Summers P, Kyei A, Bergfeld W. Central centrifugal cicatricial alopecia—an approach to diagnosis and management. Int J Dermatol 2011;50(12):1457–64.

23. Callender VD, Wright DR, Davis EC, et al. Hair breakage as a presenting sign of early or occult central centrifugal cicatricial alopecia: clinicopathologic findings in 9 patients. Arch Dermatol 2012;148(9): 1047–52.

24. Miteva M, Tosti A. Hair and scalp dermatoscopy. J Am Acad Dermatol 2012;67(5):1040–8.

25. Mubki T, Rudnicka L, Olszewska M, et al. Evaluation and diagnosis of the hair loss patient: part II. Trichoscopic and laboratory evaluations. J Am Acad Dermatol 2014;71(3):431.e1–11.

Infectious Disease Practice Gaps in Dermatology

Shelby Hopp, BS[a], Tyler L. Quest, MD[b],
Karolyn A. Wanat, MD[c],*

KEYWORDS

- Infectious disease • Dermatology • Practice gaps • Antibiotic therapy

KEY POINTS

- Infectious disease practice gaps in dermatology involve the inappropriate use of antibiotics in atopic dermatitis and acne vulgaris, in the treatment of skin and soft tissue infections, and onychomycosis.
- The use of imiquimod with molluscum contagiosum has been demonstrated as ineffective in unpublished clinical trials and has potential risk for adverse effects.
- Risk of infections related to biological immunosuppressive medications and rates of vaccination are important considerations when choosing therapy and for dermatology education and practice today.
- Bedside diagnostics for diagnosing common infections is an essential component of dermatology training that can be helpful in future practice.

INTRODUCTION

Infectious disease is an essential part of dermatology education with infections being a common presenting sign to dermatologists among all age groups.[1] Furthermore, a recent investigation into outpatient prescribing of antibiotics revealed that dermatologists prescribe more antibiotics per provider in the outpatient setting than any other specialty with an average of 724 antibiotic prescriptions per provider per year.[2] Increased attention and focus on antimicrobial stewardship is necessary in order to help minimize unnecessary antimicrobial resistance. Prolonged duration and increased use of antibiotics in patients increase the likelihood of colonization with resistant organisms.[3]

This article highlights different educational and practice gaps in infectious diseases as they pertain to dermatology. These gaps include the use of antibiotics in relation to atopic dermatitis and acne vulgaris, treatment of skin and soft tissue infection (SSTI), and diagnosing and treating onychomycosis. In addition, the use of imiquimod for molluscum contagiosum, risk of infections related to immunosuppressive medications and rates of vaccination, and the use of bedside diagnostics for diagnosing common infections were explored.

ORAL ANTIBIOTICS FOR TREATMENT OF ATOPIC DERMATITIS
Background

Atopic individuals are predisposed to skin infections secondary to a compromised physical barrier, diminished immune regulation, and impaired antimicrobial peptide production. *Staphylococcus*

Disclosure Statement: No financial disclosures or conflicts of interest.
[a] Carver College of Medicine, University of Iowa, Iowa City, IA 52242, USA; [b] Department of Dermatology, University of Iowa Hospitals and Clinics, 200 Hawkins Drive, Iowa City, IA 52242, USA; [c] Department of Dermatology, Pathology and Infectious Disease, University of Iowa Hospitals and Clinics, and VA Medical Center, 200 Hawkins Drive, Iowa City, IA 52242, USA
* Corresponding author. Department of Dermatology, Pathology, Infectious Disease, University of Iowa Hospitals and Clinics and VA Medical Center, 200 Hawkins Drive, Iowa City, IA 52242.
E-mail address: karolyn-wanat@uiowa.edu

Dermatol Clin 34 (2016) 281–289
http://dx.doi.org/10.1016/j.det.2016.02.004
0733-8635/16/$ – see front matter

aureus colonization occurs in greater than 90% of patients and triggers multiple inflammatory cascades.[4,5] Recent studies have shown that S. aureus may be not only a complication of atopic dermatitis but also an important factor in the initiation of inflammation.[6] Besides bleach baths and intranasal mupirocin, no other topical antistaphylococcal treatment has been shown to be clinically beneficial.[5,7] Furthermore, the evidence to support the use of oral antibiotics is lacking, and quantitative bacterial changes do not translate into clinical improvement. Systemic antibiotics reduce the colony count of Staphylococcus spp., but antigens may persist for prolonged periods and counts may return to previous levels within days to weeks.[4,5] Based on a recent investigation, improvement is seen in children with methicillin-resistant S. aureus (MRSA) when treated with cephalexin and other standard therapies, even when the organism was resistant to the antibiotic, suggesting that systemic antibiotics may not be necessary in secondarily impetiginized atopic dermatitis. MRSA is also reported to be more problematic in children with multiple antibiotic exposures.[8,9] A rising incidence of MRSA has also been noted in a pediatric population and is associated with antibiotic use.[10] Gong and colleagues[9] also noted that an antibiotic-corticosteroid combination and corticosteroid alone both gave adequate therapeutic effect in eczema and in atopic dermatitis, and both reduced colonization by S. aureus.

Best Practice

Antimicrobial therapy should only be considered in patients with atopic dermatitis when there is clinical evidence of infection and should be used in conjunction with other standard treatments.

Current Practice

The current practice may include the use oral and topical antibiotics as a standard treatment in patients with moderate to severe atopic dermatitis.

Practice Gap

The practice gap includes the overuse of topical and systemic antimicrobial therapy in atopic dermatitis with an underemphasis of other standard therapies, including topical corticosteroids, when there is no evidence of secondary impetiginization.

Educational Gap

The educational gap includes the use of antibiotics in atopic dermatitis without clinical evidence of infection (medical knowledge, system-based practice, patient care, professionalism).

Barriers

Barriers include provider beliefs that topical and systemic antibiotics are necessary in moderate to severe atopic dermatitis and a hesitancy to use topical steroids when there is evidence of secondary impetiginization.

TREATMENT OF COMMON SKIN AND SOFT TISSUE INFECTIONS IN THE OUTPATIENT DERMATOLOGY PRACTICE
Background

Common SSTIs resulting from Staphylococcal spp. and Streptococcal spp. infection include furuncles, carbuncles, abscesses, and cellulitis. Antimicrobial selection and duration of treatment often vary by provider. The Infectious Disease Society of America has provided clear guidelines to assist in diagnosis and treatment.[11] Guidelines indicate that incision and drainage alone are considered therapeutic for uncomplicated furuncles or abscesses, although antibiotics often are prescribed. For practicing dermatologists, knowledge of this practice is important because bacterial infections may comprise 20% of any dermatology practice.

Best Practice

Warm compresses with consideration of incision and drainage is recommended for uncomplicated furuncles or abscesses. Culture should be obtained with incision and drainage of a suspected furuncle and drainage of other purulent lesions. Systemic antimicrobial therapy is recommended with associated cellulitis, comorbidities, systemic signs of infection, or inadequate response to therapy.[11] Systemic antimicrobials and culture are not necessary with inflamed epidermal inclusion cysts. For cellulitis, if treatment is indicated in the outpatient setting, therapy for purulent cellulites should be directed toward MRSA. In nonpurulent cellulitis, therapy should be directed to β-hemolytic Streptococci spp. and methicillin-sensitive S. aureus (MSSA). Recommended duration of antimicrobial therapy is 5 to 6 days with longer courses if infection has not improved[11,12] (**Table 1**).

Current Practice

Current practice may include using antibiotics in the treatment of uncomplicated furuncles and extended and broad-spectrum therapy in uncomplicated cellulitis.

Practice Gap

The practice gap includes the overuse of systemic antimicrobials in settings where antimicrobial

Table 1
Recommended antimicrobial therapy and treatment duration for skin diseases and skin and soft tissue infections

Disease	Organism	Primary Antibiotics[11]	Duration of Therapy	Practice/Educational Gaps
Acne	*P acnes*	Tetracyclines, macrolides, topical clindamycin	3–6 mo	Extended durations, use of nonrecommended antibiotics
Atopic dermatitis	*S. aureus*	Bleach baths, intranasal mupirocin	—	Routine use of oral antimicrobial therapy
Impetigo	*S. aureus/S pyogenes*	Mupirocin, retapamulin, cephalexin, dicloxacillin, clindamycin, amoxicillin-clavulanate	Topical therapy: 5 d Oral therapy: 7 d	Extended durations
MSSA SSTI	*S. aureus*	Nafcillin, oxacillin, cefazolin, clindamycin, cephalexin, doxycycline, minocycline, trimethoprim-sulfamethoxazole	5 d in uncomplicated and if improving	Extended durations, broad spectrum antibiotics
MRSA SSTI	*S. aureus*	Vancomycin, linezolid, clindamycin, daptomycin, ceftaroline, doxycycline, minocycline, trimethoprim-sulfamethoxazole	5 d in uncomplicated and if improving	—
Nonpurulent SSTI	*Streptococcal*	Penicillin, clindamycin, nafcillin, cefazolin, penicillin VK, cephalexin	5 d in uncomplicated and if improving	Extended durations, difficulty in distinguishing purulent from nonpurulent, therapy directed at *Staphylococcus* spp.

Necrotizing infections	*S pyogenes, S. aureus, Clostridium perfringens, V vulnificus, A hydrophilia*	Surgical inspection/debridement
		Monomicrobial
		  S pyogenes: penicillin PLUS clindamycin
		  Clostridial sp: penicillin PLUS clindamycin
		  V vulnificus: doxycycline PLUS ceftazidime
		  A hydrophilia: doxycycline PLUS ciprofloxacin
		Polymicrobial:
		  Vancomycin PLUS piperacillin/tazobactam
			—	Essential to recognize signs and symptoms of necrotizing infections

Abbreviations: A hydrophilia, Aeromonas hydrophilia; *P acnes,* Propionibacterium acnes; *S pyogenes,* Streptococcus pyogenes; *V vulnificus,* Vibrio vulnificus.

Adapted from Stevens DL, Bisno AL, Chambers HF, et al. Practice guidelines for the diagnosis and management of skin and soft tissue infections: 2014 update by the Infectious Diseases Society of America. Clin Infect Dis 2014;59(2):e10–52; and Hepburn MJ, Dooley DP, Skidmore PJ, et al. Comparison of short-course (5 days) and standard (10 days) treatment for uncomplicated cellulitis. Arch Intern Med 2004;164(15):1669–74.

therapy is not indicated or the duration could be limited to 5 to 6 days.

Educational Gap

The educational gap includes the use of systemic antimicrobials in uncomplicated furuncles, inflamed epidermal inclusion cysts, and extended duration therapy for uncomplicated infections (medical knowledge, system-based practice, patient care, professionalism).

Barriers

Barriers include a reluctance to decrease the duration of antimicrobial therapy; current practices of routine use of antimicrobial therapy with inflamed epidermoid cysts; and clinical uncertainty regarding purulent versus nonpurulent cellulitis.

ANTIBIOTIC USE IN ACNE AND PROPOSED COURSE
Background

Acne is a disease of the pilosebaceous unit that affects almost all people aged 15 to 17 years and is moderate to severe in approximately 15% to 20%. There is notable variation in therapeutic regimens with numerous treatment options available including topical and oral antibiotics.[13] In a recent survey of pediatricians, almost one-third of providers self-rated knowledge of and confidence in prescribing according to the guidelines as "poor." After attending an educational session, significantly more providers selected a regimen for moderate acne that used retinoids and benzoyl peroxide. Furthermore, although 6% of providers inappropriately used antibiotics preintervention, no providers made these errors at 3 months.[14] Topical antibiotics and benzoyl peroxide are indicated in patients with mild to moderate inflammatory acne with systemic antibiotics reserved for moderate to severe acne. Systemic antibiotics exhibit their effects via inhibition of bacterial lipase, downregulating inflammatory cytokines, preventing neutrophil chemotaxis, and inhibiting matrix metalloproteinases.[15] There is no conclusive evidence that oral antibiotics are more effective than topical preparations for mild to moderate facial acne.[13] Furthermore, antibiotics are frequently prescribed without topical retinoid therapy, possibility as a result of tolerability or issues related to cost and insurance coverage[14,16–18]; this leads to prolonged duration of antimicrobial therapy and decreased efficacy of treatment.

Best Practice

Choice of antibiotic therapy should be based on side-effect profile, cost, and antibiotic-resistance profiles with preferred agents being tetracycline and derivatives. Published guidelines suggest oral antibiotic courses should be limited to 3 to 6 months and discontinued if an individual does not respond. There is no evidence that increasing dose or frequency increases efficacy.[19] Antibiotics should not be used as monotherapy and should be combined with topical retinoids and benzoyl peroxide. Finally, concomitant use of oral and topical therapy with chemically dissimilar antibiotics should be avoided.[14,16–18,20]

Current Practice

In a recent study comparing the duration of oral antibiotic use in acne with recent guidelines, it was shown that the average course duration was 129 days, and most courses were less than 9 months.[21] Although duration of antibiotic appears to be decreasing, many courses still exceeded 6 months, leaving an opportunity for reduced antibiotic use and potential cost savings.[21] Furthermore, topical and oral antibiotics are often prescribed as monotherapy, without concomitant topical retinoid, which contributes to prolonged durations.

Practice and Educational Gap

The practice and educational gap includes the extended courses of antibiotics (>6 months) and use of antibiotics without the use of a concomitant retinoid in acne vulgaris (medical knowledge, system-based practice, patient care, professionalism).

Barriers

Barriers include a patient and provider reluctance to discontinue antibiotic therapy, worsening of acne off of antimicrobial therapy, and intolerance to topical retinoid therapy.

ORAL ANTIFUNGAL USE IN NAIL FUNGUS WITHOUT CONFIRMATION OF FUNGAL INFECTION
Background

Onychodystrophy can result from numerous causes, including inflammatory disorders and fungal infection. Onychomycosis is the most common disease of the nail unit in adults but can be often confused clinically with other nail diseases. Patient safety should be considered, and failure to diagnose accurately may result in administration of an unwarranted long-term antimycotic therapy with potential side effects.[22] Conventional diagnostic techniques have proven to be of low sensitivity and specificity.

Best Practice

Confirmation of onychomycosis is recommended before systemic medications are prescribed because prolonged courses are necessary to treat nail disease. Although more research is needed to reach a consensus of the best and most cost-effective test for onychomycosis diagnosis, confirmation with one of the currently available methods should occur before treatment with an antifungal is initiated.

Existing methods for appropriate diagnosing onychomycosis include potassium hydroxide (KOH) preparation, culture of specimens, and histologic sections stained with periodic acid–Schiff or Gomori methenamine silver. Each test has its own advantages and disadvantages, and there is no current conclusive evidence for one optimal test. Other newer tests include molecular diagnostic techniques, including polymerase chain reaction assays.

Current Practice

Many practitioners empirically treat nail dystrophy as onychomycosis, trusting a clinical examination as sufficient for diagnosis and treatment, which can result drug-related risk exposure without concrete evidence of fungal infection, increased medication cost, and ineffective treatment.[23]

Practice Gap

Dermatologists prescribe oral antifungals for assumed onychomycosis before confirmation of the diagnosis (medical knowledge, system-based practice).

Educational Gap

The educational gap includes the treatment of onychomycosis in dermatology residency training without confirmation of fungal infection (medical knowledge, system-based practice).

Barriers

Barriers include a continued treatment based on clinical suspicion despite recommendations.

USE OF IMIQUIMOD FOR MOLLUSCUM CONTAGIOSUM IN CHILDREN
Background

Molluscum contagiosum is a common childhood infection that is often self-limited but frequently treated to help prevent further spread and subsequent scarring. Early trials suggested possible benefit with imiquimod treatment.[24,25] Two large randomized control trials have failed to show improvement with imiquimod compared with control vehicle; however, these trials have not been published.[26–28] A prior publication has noted that in these studies, approximately 25% of both imiquimod- and vehicle-treated children cleared their infection after 18 weeks. These data also demonstrated that children treated with imiquimod were also more likely to experience adverse reactions, including application site reaction, otitis media, leukopenia, lymphadenopathy, and conjunctivitis.[26–28]

Best Practice

The use of imiquimod in molluscum contagiosum is not currently recommended because of a lack of improvement observed in clinical trials and potential adverse events.

Current Practice

Imiquimod is currently used as a treatment for molluscum contagiosum. In a 2009 survey of health care providers regarding treatment of molluscum contagiosum, 67% of dermatologists reported prescribing imiquimod.[29–31]

Educational and Practice Gap

The educational and practice gap includes the use of imiquimod as an accepted treatment in dermatology education and practice. Katz and Swetman[26] noted "no major online references or textbooks—or even a Cochrane Collaboration systematic review of treatments for molluscum contagiosum—mentioned the 2 randomized control trials" (medical knowledge).

Barriers

Barriers include an ongoing belief that imiquimod is a useful therapeutic entity based on insufficient inclusion of current medical knowledge in dermatology training.

VACCINATION STATUS AND RISK OF INFECTION WITH BIOLOGICAL IMMUNOSUPPRESSANTS
Background

Serious infections are a rare outcome of biological immunosuppressive therapy and are therefore a difficult outcome to investigate. Multiple meta-analysis and biological registries have shown a range of data in regards to serious infection (SI). In patients with rheumatoid arthritis, a systematic review of 9 randomized controlled trials in 2006 found a doubling of the rate of SI, whereas 2 later meta-analyses showed no significantly increased risk, although they could not rule out a clinically important increase.[32–34] A recent meta-analysis from 106 trials of biological therapy in patients with rheumatoid arthritis found an increased risk in all patients but did not identify an increased risk in comparison to methotrexate in disease-modifying antirheumatic drug-naive patients.[32–34] The Psoriasis Longitudinal Assessment and Registry noted cumulative unadjusted rates of SI in the overall population were 0.83, 1.47, 1.97, and 2.49 per 100 patient-years for the ustekinumab, etanercept, adalimumab, and infliximab cohorts, respectively.[35] A higher risk of infection with adalimumab and infliximab compared with nonmethotrexate and nonbiological therapies has been shown, whereas the risk of SI is uncertain with the use of etanercept and ustekinumab and has not been conclusively demonstrated. An individual patient's comorbidities and risk factors are especially relevant in regards to risk of SI, and modifiable risk factors should be addressed before initiation of therapy[32–35] (Table 2).

Best Practice

An individualized assessment of comorbidities is more important than the specific therapy's risk of SI when selecting biological immunosuppressive therapy. Focusing on reducing the individual risk factor is an important aspect in decreasing the risk of infection. The risk of infection appears to be increased with adalimumab and infliximab, whereas an increased risk has not been clearly shown with etanercept and ustekinumab. Immunization status and need for prophylaxis should also be addressed (see Table 2).

Current Practice

Current practice emphasizes patient counseling toward the rate of increased infection with biological immunosuppressive therapy without placing equal attention on modifiable risk factors and vaccination status.

Practice Gap

The overall risk of immunosuppressive agents is not clearly understood, and individual comorbidities are not prioritized in regards to decreasing the risk of infection. Vaccination before initiation of immunosuppressants is advised. Therapy with low-dose methotrexate (<0.4 mg/kg/wk), azathioprine ($\leq$3.0 mg/kg/d), or 6-mercaptopurine ($\leq$1.5 mg/kg/d) is often misconceived as a contraindication to zoster vaccination.[36]

Educational Gap

The educational gap includes the emphasis on the increased risk of infection with biological therapy, whereas modifiable risks and vaccinations are underemphasized (medical knowledge, patient care).

USE OF BEDSIDE DIAGNOSTIC TESTS
Background

Bedside testing can help facilitate arriving at a diagnosis quickly, allowing for treatment to be initiated. Common bedside tests include KOH preparation, Tzanck smear, mineral oil preparation, and Gram stain. Although these tests are quick and relatively easy to perform, residents may not receive training on how to perform and when to perform these tests, and practicing dermatologists may lose their skills without use.[37]

Best Practice

The KOH preparation is used to diagnose fungal and yeast infections. This process begins by collecting the specimen, placing the specimen on a microscope slide, applying KOH solution, and waiting at least 5 minutes before reading the slide to allow for digestion of the keratin. The Tzanck smear is useful for diagnosis of herpetic lesions, but may also be more widely applied to diagnosis of pustular diseases, cutaneous infection, vesiculobullous disease, and nonmelanoma skin cancer.[38] A sample is collected by scraping the base of a fresh blister; the scrapings are then smeared onto a slide and allowed to air dry. Wright-Giemsa stain is used followed by rinsing with sterile water. A mineral oil preparation is useful in the diagnosis of scabies and Demodex. Several drops of mineral oil are placed onto a slide and then the blade is dipped into the mineral oil before scraping the sample lesion to allow the debris to collect in the mineral oil.[37,39,40] Clinical laboratory improvement amendments (CLIA) are required to perform these tests for purposes of patient care.

Current Practice

These quick bedside tests may be substituted by biopsies, cultures, or more detailed diagnostic techniques, which increase cost and can delay treatment.

Practice Gap

The practice gap includes the limited use of bedside diagnostic testing in dermatology practice secondary to clinic flow or need for CLIA certification.

Educational Gap

There is a lack of training on proper use and utility of these bedside tests during dermatology

Table 2
Considerations when beginning/continuing iatrogenic immunosuppression

Best Practice	Best Practice Strategies	Barriers	Strategies to Overcome Barriers
Screen for risk factors	Immunosuppressive illnesses, pertinent history (blood transfusion, high-risk sexual activity, travel, PPD test, nutritional deficiency)	Chronic illnesses that are difficult to treat; provider resources	Multidisciplinary support from primary care and appropriate specialists and frequent follow-up
Screening for existing or latent infections	Hepatitis B, hepatitis C, HIV, tuberculosis, Strongyloides (from endemic areas), some investigators recommend consideration of systemic fungal infections on individualized basis if from endemic areas or risk factors (cryptococcosis, histoplasmosis, coccidioidomycosis, blastomycosis, paracoccidioidomycosis)	Knowledge of tests to order for patients of certain populations	Education on tests to order for systemic medications
Prophylaxis	Pneumocystis pneumonia in patients treated with TNF-α inhibitors if they are also receiving high-dose glucocorticoids or other intensive immunosuppression, patients on 3 immunosuppressive agents, patients with other forms of immunocompromise	Uncertainty of need for prophylaxis based on different recommendations	The use of pneumocystis prophylaxis if patients are on TNF-α inhibitors and other intensive immunosuppression or 3 immunosuppressive agents
Up-to-date immunizations	Influenza, pneumococcus, herpes zoster, tetanus/diphtheria	Lack of addressing immunization status	Addressing immunization status before initiation; establishing immunization templates before prescribing
Patient education	Hand washing, avoid high-risk exposures, early signs/symptoms of infections	Lack of patient counseling	Routine discussion at every clinic visit
Monitor at follow-up visits	Look for impetiginization and colonization of HSV, Candida, and Staphylococcus; review of systems; laboratory monitoring	—	—

Abbreviations: HIV, human immunodeficiency virus; PPD, purified protein derivative; TNF-α, tumor necrosis factor-α.
Adapted from Lehman JS, Wetter DA, Davis MDP, et al. Anticipating and preventing infection in patients treated with immunosuppressive medications for dermatologic indications: a dermatologist's checklist. J Am Acad Dermatol 2014;71(4):e125–6; and Rodriguez M, Fishman JA. Prevention of infection due to Pneumocystis spp. in human immunodeficiency virus-negative immunocompromised patients. Clin Microbiol Rev 2004;17(4):770.

residency training (medical knowledge, practice-based learning).

Barriers

Barriers include limited resources available to provide training and resources devoted to maintaining a CLIA-certified laboratory with official training programs.

REFERENCES

1. Landis ET, Davis SA, Taheri A, et al. Top dermatologic diagnoses by age. Dermatol Online J 2014; 20(4):22368.
2. Hicks LA, Bartoces MG, Roberts RM, et al. US outpatient antibiotic prescribing variation according to geography, patient population, and provider specialty in 2011. Clin Infect Dis 2015;60(9):1308–16.
3. Dellit TH, Owens RC, McGowan JE, et al. Infectious Diseases Society of America and the Society for Healthcare Epidemiology of America Guidelines for developing an institutional program to enhance antimicrobial stewardship. Clin Infect Dis 2007;44(2):159–77.
4. Sidbury R, Tom WL, Bergman JN, et al. Guidelines of care for the management of atopic dermatitis: Section 4. Prevention of disease flares and use of adjunctive therapies and approaches. J Am Acad Dermatol 2014;71(6):1218–33.
5. Bath-Hextall FJ, Birnie AJ, Ravenscroft JC, et al. Interventions to reduce Staphylococcus aureus in the management of atopic eczema: an updated Cochrane Review. Br J Dermatol 2010;163(1):12–26.
6. Kobayashi T, Glatz M, Horiuchi K, et al. Dysbiosis and Staphylococcus aureus colonization drives inflammation in atopic dermatitis. Immunity 2015; 42(4):756–66.
7. Eichenfield LF, Tom WL, Berger TG, et al. Guidelines of care for the management of atopic dermatitis: Section 2. Management and treatment of atopic dermatitis with topical therapies. J Am Acad Dermatol 2014;71(1):116–32.
8. Travers JB, Kozman A, Yao Y, et al. Treatment outcomes of secondarily impetiginized pediatric atopic dermatitis lesions and the role of oral antibiotics. Pediatr Dermatol 2012;29(3):289–96.
9. Gong JQ, Lin L, Lin T, et al. Skin colonization by Staphylococcus aureus in patients with eczema and atopic dermatitis and relevant combined topical therapy: a double-blind multicentre randomized controlled trial. Br J Dermatol 2006;155(4):680–7.
10. Schneider-Lindner V, Quach C, Hanley JA, et al. Antibacterial drugs and the risk of community-associated methicillin-resistant Staphylococcus aureus in children. Arch Pediatr Adolesc Med 2011;165(12):1107–14.
11. Stevens DL, Bisno AL, Chambers HF, et al. Practice guidelines for the diagnosis and management of skin and soft tissue infections: 2014 Update by the Infectious Diseases Society of America. Clin Infect Dis 2014;59(2):e10–52.
12. Hepburn MJ, Dooley DP, Skidmore PJ, et al. Comparison of short-course (5 days) and standard (10 days) treatment for uncomplicated cellulitis. Arch Intern Med 2004;164(15):1669–74.
13. Williams HC, Dellavalle RP, Garner S. Acne vulgaris. Lancet 2012;379(9813):361–72.
14. Davis SA, Sandoval LF, Gustafson CJ, et al. Treatment of preadolescent acne in the United States: an analysis of nationally representative data. Pediatr Dermatol 2013;30(6):689–94.
15. Das S, Reynolds R. Recent advances in acne pathogenesis: implications for therapy. Am J Clin Dermatol 2014;15(6):479–88.
16. Straight CE, Lee YH, Liu G, et al. Duration of oral antibiotic therapy for the treatment of adult acne: a retrospective analysis investigating adherence to guideline recommendations and opportunities for cost-savings. J Am Acad Dermatol 2015;72(5): 822–7.
17. Thiboutot D, Gollnick H, Bettoli V, et al. New insights into the management of acne: an update from the Global Alliance to Improve Outcomes in Acne Group. J Am Acad Dermatol 2009;60(5 Suppl 1): S1–50.
18. Gollnick H, Cunliffe W, Berson D, et al. Management of acne: a report from a global alliance to improve outcomes in acne. J Am Acad Dermatol 2003; 49(Suppl 1):S1–37.
19. Nast A, Dréno B, Bettoli V, et al. European evidence-based (S3) guidelines for the treatment of acne. J Eur Acad Dermatol Venereol 2012;26:1–29.
20. Eichenfield LF, Krakowski AC, Piggott C, et al. Evidence-based recommendations for the diagnosis and treatment of pediatric acne. Pediatrics 2013; 131(Suppl 3):S163–86.
21. Lee YH, Liu G, Thiboutot DM, et al. A retrospective analysis of the duration of oral antibiotic therapy for the treatment of acne among adolescents: investigating practice gaps and potential cost-savings. J Am Acad Dermatol 2014;71(1):70–6.
22. Grover C, Reddy BS, Chaturvedi KU. Onychomycosis and the diagnostic significance of nail biopsy. J Dermatol 2003;30:116–22.
23. Stewart CL, Rubin AI. Update: nail unit dermatopathology. Dermatol Ther 2012;25(6):551–68.
24. Al-Mutairi N, Al-Doukhi A, Al-Farrag S, et al. Comparative study on the efficacy, safety, and acceptability of imiquimod 5% cream versus cryotherapy for molluscum contagiosum in children. Pediatr Dermatol 2010;27(4):388–94.
25. Theos A, Cummins R, Silverberg N, et al. Effectiveness of imiquimod cream 5% for treating childhood molluscum contagiosum in a double-blind, randomized pilot trial. Cutis 2004;74(2):134–8, 141–2.

26. Katz KA, Swetman GL. Imiquimod, molluscum, and the need for a better "best pharmaceuticals for children" act. Pediatrics 2013;132(1):1–3.

27. Aldara (imiquimod) cream for topical use. Dailymed. Available at: http://dailymed.nlm.nih.gov/dailymed/lookup.cfm?setid=7fccca4e-fb8f-42b8-9555-8f78a5804ed3. Accessed October 15, 2015.

28. Papadopoulos E. Clinical executive summary [Imiquimod]. 2006. Available at: http://www.fda.gov/downloads/Drugs/DevelopmentApprovalProcess/DevelopmentResources/UCM162961.pdf. Accessed October 15, 2015.

29. Katz K. Dermatologists, imiquimod, and treatment of molluscum contagiosum in children: righting wrongs. JAMA Dermatol 2015;151(2):125–6.

30. Hughes C, Damon IK, Reynolds MG. Understanding U.S. healthcare providers' practices and experiences with molluscum contagiosum. PLoS One 2013;8(10):e76948.

31. Katz K. Imiquimod is not an effective drug for molluscum contagiosum. Lancet Infect Dis 2014;14(5):372–3.

32. Dixon WG. Rheumatoid arthritis: biological drugs and risk of infection. Lancet 2015;386(9990):224–5.

33. Dao KH, Herbert M, Habal N, et al. Nonserious infections: should there be cause for serious concerns? Rheum Dis Clin North Am 2012;38(4):707–25.

34. Singh JA, Cameron C, Noorbaloochi S, et al. Risk of serious infection in biological treatment of patients with rheumatoid arthritis: a systematic review and meta-analysis. Lancet 2015;386(9990):258–65.

35. Kalb RE, Fiorentino DF, Lebwohl MG, et al. Risk of serious infection with biologic and systemic treatment of psoriasis: results from the psoriasis longitudinal assessment and registry (PSOLAR). JAMA Dermatol 2015;151(9):961–9.

36. CDC. Conditions commonly misperceived as contraindications to vaccination. 2012. Available at: http://www.cdc.gov/vaccines/recs/vac-admin/contraindications-misconceptions.htm. 2015. Accessed October 15, 2015.

37. Bronfenbrener RM. Stains and smears: resident guide to bedside diagnostic testing. Cutis 2014; 94(6):E29–30.

38. Kelly B, Shimoni T. Reintroducing the Tzanck smear. Am J Clin Dermatol 2009;10(3):141–52.

39. Gupta L, Singhi M. Tzanck smear: a useful diagnostic tool. Indian J Dermatol Venereol Leprol 2005;71(4):295–9.

40. Ruocco E, Baroni A, Donnarumma G, et al. Diagnostic procedures in dermatology. Clin Dermatol 2011;29(5):548–56.

Practice and Educational Gaps in Abnormal Pigmentation

Tasneem F. Mohammad, MD, Iltefat H. Hamzavi, MD*

KEYWORDS

- Dyschromia • Postinflammatory hyperpigmentation • Melasma • Vitiligo • Treatment
- Hyperpigmentation • Hypopigmentation • Education

KEY POINTS

- Dyschromia is one of the most common diagnoses in dermatology, yet there are significant educational and practice gaps in this area.
- The main educational and practice gaps in melasma and postinflammatory hyperpigmentation include alternative or adjunct therapies to hydroquinone and lack of exposure to a variety of skin tones.
- The main educational and practice gaps in vitiligo include underutilization and customization of phototherapy, use of agents for stabilization of progressive disease, and surgical treatment of vitiligo.
- Residency programs need to address educational gaps in disorders of pigmentation to prevent educational gaps from becoming practice gaps.

INTRODUCTION

Dyschromia refers to abnormal pigmentation of the skin or nails, including numerous conditions that cause both hyperpigmentation and hypopigmentation. It is one of the most common diagnoses in dermatology, especially in individuals with skin of color. From 1993 to 2010, there were approximately 24.7 million office visits made to dermatology practices for the management of dyschromia.[1] Despite the high prevalence of dyschromia in the general population, there is a disconnect between the occurrence of this condition and the resources directed toward its management. As such, it is important to define the standard of care for abnormal pigmentation, more specifically, postinflammatory hyperpigmentation (PIH), melasma, and vitiligo, as well as address clinical and educational gaps that may lead to substandard practices.

GOLD STANDARD
Melasma/Postinflammatory Hyperpigmentation

Melasma is a condition characterized by irregularly shaped hyperpigmented patches most commonly located in a centrofacial, malar, or mandibular pattern. Depending on the location of pigment deposition, melasma can be characterized as epidermal, dermal, or mixed type, with worse prognosis associated with dermal pigmentation. Pigment location can be determined by examination under a Wood lamp, with epidermal pigment

Disclosures: Dr I.H. Hamzavi is an investigator for Estee Lauder, Ferndale, and Allergan and has received equipment from Johnson and Johnson. Dr T.F. Mohammad is a sub-investigator for Estee Lauder, Ferndale, and Allergan.
Department of Dermatology, Henry Ford Hospital, 3031 West Grand Boulevard, Suite 800, Detroit, MI, USA
* Corresponding author. Department of Dermatology, Henry Ford Hospital, 3031 West Grand Boulevard, Suite 800, Detroit, MI 48202.
E-mail address: ihamzav1@hfhs.org

Dermatol Clin 34 (2016) 291–301
http://dx.doi.org/10.1016/j.det.2016.02.005
0733-8635/16/$ – see front matter © 2016 Elsevier Inc. All rights reserved.

derm.theclinics.com

becoming accentuated under illumination. Melasma is often associated with UV exposure, genetic predisposition, and hormonal changes, such as pregnancy or the initiation of oral contraceptive pills (OCPs). PIH occurs when cutaneous inflammation leads to increased pigmentation in the dermis or epidermis. Several conditions are capable of inducing PIH, such as atopic dermatitis, acne, medication reactions, and procedure-related inflammation. Hyperpigmentation develops in the same area as preceding inflammation and occurs more commonly in skin types III–VI.[2]

Evaluation of melasma is performed using the Melasma Area and Severity Index, or MASI, score. This evaluation involves adding the severity ratings for darkness and homogeneity, which are then multiplied by the numerical value given for 4 facial areas, including the forehead, chin, and left and right malar regions, and the percentage involvement of each area. A modified MASI score, which removes the homogeneity parameter, has subsequently been created. Clinical photography is also important in following this condition over time.[3] The MelasQoL is a scale that assesses the impact of melasma on quality of life (QoL).[4] The only validated outcome measure for evaluation of PIH is the Postacne Hyperpigmentation Index. Scoring is based on median lesion size, intensity, and number of lesions.[5] A PIH Investigator's Global Assessment scale has also been developed at Henry Ford Hospital to characterize the intensity of hyperpigmentation.[6] Serial photography is also important in monitoring progression and treatment response. Currently, no validated quality-of-life measure specific to PIH exists.

The first step in treatment of both melasma and PIH is the avoidance of causative factors. In patients with melasma, those currently taking OCPs should switch to an alternate form of birth control.[7] With regards to PIH, treatment of the underlying condition causing cutaneous inflammation is imperative. In both instances, photoprotection is critical because UV exposure can exacerbate hyperpigmentation.[3] Although most broad-spectrum chemical sunscreens provide protection against both UV-A and UV-B wavelengths, they are not effective against visible light. Visible light has been shown to induce production of reactive oxygen species (ROS) in addition to proinflammatory cytokines, and matrix metalloproteinase 1.[8] A study performed by Mahmoud and colleagues[9] showed that exposure to visible light induced pigmentation in skin types IV–VI, which was darker and more sustained than pigmentation caused by UV exposure. Physical sunscreens, such as iron oxide, provide coverage against the visible light spectrum and are often present in commercially available make-up products. Use of tinted sunscreen containing iron oxide in patients with melasma showed a smaller increase in MASI scores over time compared with patients using the same sunscreen without iron oxide.[10] Another study comparing the use of a visible light-UV sunscreen and hydroquinone to UV-only sunscreen with hydroquinone showed greater increases in MASI scores with the UV-only sunscreen and hydroquinone combination.[11] There is a paucity of literature regarding the effect of physical sunscreens in PIH, which is an area that needs to be addressed in future studies.

With respect to topical therapies, hydroquinone is the mainstay of treatment. Inhibition of tyrosinase, the enzyme responsible for converting dihydrophenylalanine to melanin, is its main mechanism of action. It can be used alone, but is more effective when used in combination with a retinoid and corticosteroid, which is known as Kligman's formula.[7] However, caution is advised because use of hydroquinone has been associated with ochronosis, a blackish discoloration of the skin that is difficult to reverse.[12] Currently, there are several other lightening agents that can be used as an alternative or adjunct to hydroquinone. Examples include soy, ellagic acid, niacinamide, licorice extract, kojic acid, vitamin C, and arbutin (**Table 1**). These compounds have been shown to cause statistically significant reductions in pigmentation. Most of these alternative therapies are available as over-the-counter products.[13,14]

Currently, there are few oral therapies being used for the treatment of melasma or PIH. Most commonly used in Southeast Asia, tranexamic acid is a plasmin inhibitor that has been used to treat melasma successfully. Multiple studies have shown that oral tranexamic acid decreases MASI scores when used in both monotherapy and combination therapy. Nausea, diarrhea, menstrual irregularities, headaches, and back pain are the most commonly reported side effects. No increased risk of thromboembolic events has been noted.[4,15] This option is possible for the patient with recalcitrant melasma who has not responded to conventional therapies. Studies on the use of polypodium leucotomos extract (PLE), an oral antioxidant, for melasma have also shown improvement in MASI scores when used in conjunction with photoprotection. It has been postulated that PLE would be beneficial in treatment of PIH due to its anti-inflammatory effects, but no specific studies have been performed to investigate this theory.[16]

Chemical peels as well as light-based and laser therapy have been used in the management of melasma and PIH with varying success. Extreme caution must be used when using these modalities in skin types IV–VI because a risk of creating post-procedural PIH exists. Commonly used peels include salicylic acid, glycolic acid, Jessner solution, and TCA (trichloroacetic acid) peels. Several different lasers, such as the Q-switched 1064-nm neodymium-doped yttrium aluminum garnet (Nd:YAG) and 1550-nm erbium glass, have been used to treat melasma and PIH with varying success. An observational study of women with skin types II–V treated with micro-dermabrasion followed by Q-switched Nd:YAG and then a topical maintenance regimen showed significant clearance of hyperpigmentation that lasted for at least 6 months.[17] Fractional resurfacing has also shown improvement in MASI scores; however, recurrence is common when used as monotherapy.[18] Intense pulsed light has also been used in skin types I–III.[4]

Vitiligo

Affecting approximately 0.5% to 2% of the population worldwide, vitiligo is a condition marked by cutaneous depigmentation that can have a severe psychosocial impact on patients.[19] The cause is multifactorial, including an impaired response to oxidative stress, autoimmunity, as well as a neuro-humoral component.[20] Vitiligo is generally classified as either segmental or non-segmental, which includes several variants, including generalized vitiligo, the most common subtype. Generalized vitiligo is usually symmetric and bilateral and has a waxing and waning course. On the other hand, segmental vitiligo is typically unilateral, localized to one region, and characterized by a stable course.[21]

Evaluation of vitiligo is performed by physical examination under a Wood's lamp, with depigmented areas fluorescing. Serial photography is also necessary for monitoring responsiveness to treatment. The degree of involvement can be assessed using either the Vitiligo Area Scoring Index (VASI) or the Vitiligo European Task Force assessment (VETFa). The VASI score is calculated by multiplying involved surface area by the degree of depigmentation for 5 separate regions of the body, including the hands, feet, upper extremities, lower extremities, and the trunk. The neck and face are evaluated separately. The total values for each region are then added to give the final VASI score. In addition to taking depigmentation into account, the VETFa also includes stage and progression of disease in scoring. A comparison of these instruments shows that both are reliable in measuring the degree of depigmentation, with high levels of interobserver and intraobserver reliability.[22] To determine the psychosocial impact

of vitiligo, the VitiQoL, a validated assessment of quality of life (QoL) specific to vitiligo, can be used.[23] The Vitiligo Impact Scale-22, another validated measure of QoL specific for vitiligo, can also be used.[24]

Appropriate treatment of vitiligo is dependent on the clinical subtype (**Fig. 1**). On diagnosis of generalized vitiligo, patients should be screened for concurrent autoimmune disorders, such as hypothyroidism.[25] Photoprotection is also important because tanning of the skin leads to increased contrast with depigmented areas. Also, depigmented skin is more photosensitive than surrounding skin and koebnerization can be seen in response to sunburn.[26]

For localized regions of vitiligo, application of topical corticosteroids or calcineurin inhibitors should be initiated as monotherapy or in combination. Vitamin D analogues, although effective in treatment of psoriasis, are not as effective in vitiligo. Studies have shown some increase in repigmentation when used as an adjunct to topical corticosteroids and phototherapy. However, they are not considered first-line therapy.[27] Targeted phototherapy using narrow band ultraviolet B (NBUVB) or excimer laser is also effective in repigmenting localized lesions.[28]

Surgical treatment of discrete depigmented areas is possible for select patients with vitiligo. Good surgical candidates include those with segmental vitiligo, stable disease for at least 6 months, and lack of distal acral involvement, as distal depigmentation is associated with poor outcomes.[29] Although many surgical techniques have been described in the literature, the most effective surgical methods include split-thickness skin grafts, blister grafts, and the melanocyte keratinocyte transplant procedure (MKTP). In all 3 techniques, the recipient site is prepared by removal of the epidermis through multiple methods, including dermabrasion or CO_2 laser. Split-thickness skin grafts are obtained by removing the epidermis along with a portion of the dermis using a blade. These portions are then laid over the prepared recipient site. Blister grafts involve inducing a suction blister at the donor site and then cutting off the blister roof and transferring it to the recipient site. In MKTP, an ultrathin split-thickness skin graft is taken from the donor site and incubated with trypsin. Then, cell separation is performed to isolate the melanocytes and keratinocytes. These cells are then made into a cellular suspension that is applied to the recipient site. The benefit of this method is that larger surface areas can be treated, often at a 10:1 ratio to the donor site.[30]

For patients with generalized disease, topical therapy with corticosteroids and calcineurin

Table 1
Agents for treatment of hyperpigmentation

Ingredient	Mechanism	Products	Comments
Hydroquinone	• Inhibits tyrosinase • Inhibits synthesis of melanocyte DNA and RNA	Nadinola	• Risk of ochranosis with overuse • May require prescription depending on percentage
HQ/retinoid/CS	Retinoid: • Inhibits tyrosinase • Increases turnover of keratinocytes • Increases dispersal of keratinocyte pigment granules Corticosteroid: • Anti-inflammatory	Triluma	• First-line treatment for hyperpigmentation • Requires prescription
Azelaic acid	• Inhibits tyrosinase	• PCA Skin Pigment Bar (combination of kojic acid and azelaic acid)	• Also used in many acne and rosacea products • Available in OTC products and as a prescription product
Mequinol	• Competitive inhibitor of tyrosinase	Solage (combination product of mequinol/retinoid)	• Less irritating than hydroquinone
Kojic acid	• Inhibits tyrosinase by binding copper • Scavenger of ROS	La Roche-Posay Mela-D Pigment Control (combination of kojic acid, LHA, and glycolic acid)	• Chelation agent produced by fungi • Can be combined with glycolic acid to improve penetration and LHA to increase cellular turnover
Soy	• PAR-2 inhibitor • Suppresses melanosome transfer • Suppresses ROS	Aveeno Active Naturals Positively Radiant Neutrogena Visibly Even Daily Moisturizer	• Also has surfactant activity
N-acetylglucosamine	• Inhibits conversion of protyrosinase to tyrosinase	Olay Total Effects Tone Correcting Moisturizer (combination product with niacinamide)	• Monomeric unit of chitin, which makes up the exoskeleton of insects and crustaceans
Licorice extract	• Inhibits tyrosinase • Suppresses ROS	• Lancôme Bright Expert Dark Spot Corrector • The Body Shop Moisture White Shiso Moisture Cream	• Obtained from the root of *Glycyrrhiza glabra*

	Mechanism	Product examples	Notes
Arbutin	• Competitive inhibitor of tyrosinase	• Timeless Skin Care Skin Lightening Cream (combination of arbutin, vitamin C, kojic acid) • Skinceuticals Phyto + Botanical Gel for Hyperpigmentation (combination of arbutin, kojic acid)	• Derivative of HQ found in pears, blueberries, cranberries, and wheat
Vitamin C	• Inhibits tyrosinase through interaction with copper	• Garnier Skin Renew Clinical Dark Spot Corrector • Shiseido White Lucent Intensive Spot Targeting Serum	• Rapidly oxidized and unstable; drug delivery is important limiting factor
Niacinamide	• Inhibits melanosome transfer to keratinocytes	• L'Oreal Youth Code Dark Spot Serum Corrector • Philosophy Miracle Worker Dark Spot Corrector	• Active derivative of vitamin B3
Emblica	• Inhibits tyrosinase • Suppresses ROS	• Skinceuticals Pigment Regulator Daily High Potency Brightening Treatment (combination of emblica extract, kojic acid)	• Derived from Indian gooseberries
Lignin peroxidase	• Depolymerizes melanin	• Elure Advanced Lightening Lotion	• Enzyme derived from tree fungus
Glutathione	• Inhibits tyrosinase	• Available as OTC supplement	• Endogenously produced antioxidant
Ellagic acid	• Inhibits tyrosinase	• In combination with salicylic acid	• Also has antioxidant properties
Tumeric	• Antioxidant	• Ole Henriksen Visual Truth Eye Cream	• Also has wound-healing properties
Mulberry	• Inhibits tyrosinase	• Docteur Renaud (Paris)	—
Aloesin	• Inhibits tyrosinase	• Jan Marini Transformation Cream	• Derived from aloe vera
Green tea	• Antioxidant	• MD formulations Moisture Defense Antioxidant Hydrating Gel	—

Abbreviations: CS, corticosteroid; HQ, hydroquinone; LHA, lipohydroxy acid; OTC, over the counter.
Adapted from Refs. [2,13,14,52–55]

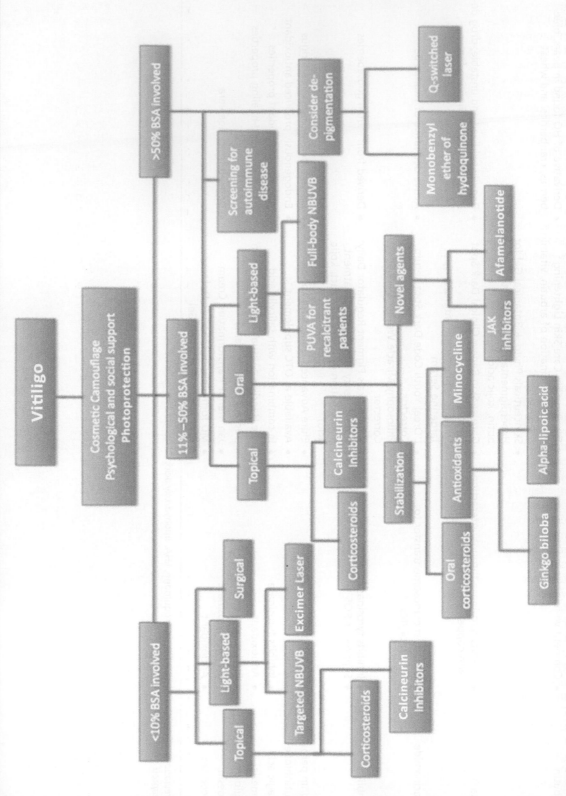

Fig. 1. Treatment of vitiligo. BSA, body surface area. (*Adapted from* Refs.[19,21,25-29,31-33,35-37,39])

inhibitors can be used. However, phototherapy should also be initiated. Psoralen and ultraviolet A (PUVA) radiation was previously the mainstay of phototherapy but it has largely been replaced with NBUVB because of a better side-effect profile and color match.[31] For patients with unstable disease, there are multiple options to halt progression. Antioxidants, such as ginkgo biloba and α-lipoic acid, are often prescribed. Patients should be warned about increased bleeding risk with ginkgo biloba. Studies on PLE in combination with phototherapy have also shown significant improvement in repigmentation.[16] Either oral corticosteroids or minocycline can be prescribed in conjunction with antioxidants to halt disease progression. Steroids can be prescribed daily or with minipulse dosing, which involves taking dexamethasone 2 consecutive days of the week for several weeks to months. Patients should be counseled about steroid side effects and told to increase dietary intake of calcium and vitamin D, or start supplementation. Prescribing bisphosphonates is a consideration for patients requiring a longer duration of therapy. When taken at a dose of 100 mg daily, minocycline has been shown to be equally effective as minipulse oral steroids in halting disease progression because of its anti-inflammatory and immunomodulatory properties.[32]

Oral immunosuppressants have been used for the treatment of vitiligo with varying success. Concurrent use of azathioprine and PUVA was shown to increase repigmentation compared with PUVA alone.[33] The combination of cyclophosphamide and dexamethasone was shown to cause repigmentation in a patient with both pemphigus vulgaris and vitiligo.[34] Another case study of 33 patients on cyclophosphamide was reported to show improvement in repigmentation in 29 patients.[25] Other immunosuppressants have been less successful. A study of 6 patients on cyclosporine showed minimal to moderate repigmentation in only one patient, whereas a study looking at the efficacy of etanercept, adalimumab, and infliximab showed no improvement in pigmentation with any of these biologics.[19] However, new molecular pathways, such as the Janus Kinase (JAK), interleukin-17, and C-X-C motif chemokine 10 (CXCL-10) pathways, are being researched and may hold the key to future therapies. Tofacitinib, a JAK-1/3 inhibitor that is US Food and Drug Administration approved for rheumatoid arthritis, was recently reported to cause repigmentation in a patient with progressive generalized vitiligo. However, clinical trials are necessary to further define the role of tofacitinib in treatment of vitiligo.[35] Afamelanotide, an α-melanocyte-stimulating hormone (α-MSH) agonist, is another novel medication that led to significant

repigmentation in combination with NBUVB phototherapy in skin types IV–VI. Although this implantable medication has been tested in a multicenter randomized clinical trial, it is not yet commercially available.[36]

Patients who do not desire medical treatment, or are not satisfied by the extent of repigmentation with therapy, can use cosmetics to camouflage their lesions. Micropigmentation, or tattooing, over areas of vitiligo is generally not recommended because of associated risks, difficulty in color matching, and fading of pigments over time.[37] Also, many flesh-colored dyes contain iron oxide, which turns black on laser-mediated tattoo removal and is cosmetically distressing for the patient and often requires extensive treatment for improvement.[38]

In patients with more than 50% of body surface area involvement, depigmentation is another option and is often done with either monobenzyl ether of hydroquinone or a Q-switched ruby laser. However, patients require psychological evaluation before proceeding. Because vitiligo can have such a profound impact on the identity and psychosocial health of a patient, it is important to assess patient's QoL and provide resources, possibly through counseling or by involvement in a support group, thereby providing patients with an environment of acceptance and understanding.[19]

Treatment of segmental vitiligo involves use of topical therapies, such as corticosteroids and calcineurin inhibitors. Targeted NBUVB phototherapy or excimer laser can also be used.[25] Although segmental vitiligo typically has a poor response to medical management, it responds very well to surgical intervention.[39]

EDUCATION IN RESIDENCY

For most dermatology residency programs, the curriculum is multifaceted, involving the review of textbooks and journals, lectures at didactics, grand rounds, and conferences, as well as clinical experience. Although most residents study a small number of established textbooks and attend major conferences, such as the American Academy of Dermatology (AAD), the quality of didactic sessions and clinical exposure to disorders of pigmentation vary. Each institution has its own area of expertise, and not all institutions have a large enough patient population with skin of color or pigmentary disorders to place an emphasis on it. Because of this variation, resident education was evaluated by performing a review of the most highly read dermatology textbooks and an evaluation of presentations given at the 2015 annual AAD meeting on melasma, PIH, and vitiligo. Texts reviewed include *Dermatology*, *Fitzpatrick's Color Atlas and Synopsis of Clinical Dermatology*, *Andrews' Diseases of the Skin: Clinical Dermatology*, *Treatment of Skin Disease*, and *Dermatology In-Review*.

Melasma/Postinflammatory Hyperpigmentation

In all of the texts reviewed, melasma was emphasized over PIH. Some texts did not even have a separate section for PIH, but included it under acne or another dermatologic condition. In most cases, hydroquinone alone or as part of a combination product was mentioned as a mainstay of therapy with azelaic acid as an alternative. Three of 5 sources mentioned photoprotection, alternatives to hydroquinone, or procedural options.[40–44]

This year at the AAD, multiple presentations were given on melasma, including updates on melasma, pathogenesis, and treatment. Advances in the treatment of pigmentary disorders, skin of color, and facial pigmentation were also addressed. A comprehensive review of cosmeceuticals that included detailed discussion of skin-lighteners and their mechanisms of action was presented as well.[45] These presentations could serve as a source of both context and information to fill in education gaps.

Vitiligo

With respect to vitiligo, all texts mentioned topical corticosteroids, calcineurin inhibitors, and phototherapy as treatment options. However, principles of phototherapy and guidelines were not discussed. Surgical techniques were mentioned, but many sources included methods that are no longer commonly used, such as punch minigrafts or dermoscopic dermal grafts. Most texts mentioned photoprotection and depigmentation, but antioxidant therapy and the psychosocial needs of patients were minimally discussed. With respect to stabilizing disease, oral minipulse therapy was mentioned in only one text as a controversial treatment, while minocycline was not discussed at all. Use of oral immunosuppressants, excluding corticosteroids, and novel molecular pathways were not reviewed either.[40,43,44,46,47]

Presentations on vitiligo at the AAD included presentations on a general and global overview of vitiligo, systemic therapies, treatment updates, surgical therapies, photoprotection, phototherapy, and the molecular pathogenesis of vitiligo. Afamelanotide, an α-MSH analogue that has been shown to increase the rate of repigmentation in patients receiving concurrent phototherapy, was also discussed.[45]

EDUCATIONAL GAPS IN RESIDENCY
Melasma/Postinflammatory Hyperpigmentation

The main educational gaps with respect to melasma and PIH are due to lack of knowledge and exposure. Currently, there is no standard guideline for treatment and maintenance therapy for these conditions. Although most residents are taught to use hydroquinone alone or as a combination product, alternative or adjunct therapies are not emphasized. Although lectures containing up-to-date information are presented at conferences, these lectures may not be attended. In terms of exposure, not all institutions have a high volume of patients presenting with a variety of skin tones. Because the appearance of erythema and dyspigmentation varies greatly between skin types and tones, residents do not learn how to treat this patient population appropriately. In addition, most patients do not have long-term follow-up or photographic records, which prevents residents from gaining an understanding of the waxing and waning course of these pigmentary disorders and the need for maintenance therapy. A study published by Nijhawan and colleagues[48] in 2008 showed that a minority of programs surveyed had a specific rotation focusing on treating skin of color, an expert in ethnic skin at their institution, or didactics given by experts in skin of color. Also, exposure to lasers and other procedural techniques may be limited at some institutions.

Vitiligo

Both lack of knowledge and exposure are responsible for educational gaps in vitiligo. The main deficits in vitiligo involve disease stabilization, surgical options, the role of systemic immunosuppression and novel pathways, and phototherapy guidelines. There is also a lack of emphasis placed on the psychosocial impact of vitiligo on patients. Stabilizing disease with therapies such as minocycline has only been described in the literature in the past few years, so institutions without a focus on vitiligo may not know about these treatment options. Vitiligo surgery is currently underperformed in the United States. Very few institutions in the United States perform vitiligo surgery, and at these locations, residents are not always required to participate as part of their curriculum. Because of a lack of strong positive results in the past, systemic immunosuppression is not given much importance during discussion of vitiligo. However, novel molecular pathways are currently being researched and will likely play a key role for future treatment. Prescription of phototherapy, especially home phototherapy, is an area of deficiency in most residency programs. According to an abstract presented at the 2015 Annual Photomedicine Society Meeting, although most third-year residents surveyed felt comfortable prescribing in-office phototherapy, less than 20% felt able to prescribe home phototherapy, leading to its underuse, although it has been shown to be comparable to in-office phototherapy.[49–51]

Solutions

To remedy the educational deficits in abnormal pigmentation, residency programs need to recognize that gaps exist and review their curriculum. Once a need for increased emphasis on these areas is acknowledged, these deficits can be remedied. Didactic sessions led by experts in skin of color, disorders of pigmentation, or vitiligo will give residents a greater understanding of the pathogenesis and treatment of these diseases. Journal clubs should have sessions dedicated to review of new literature regarding these topics, and attendance of lectures focusing on disorders of pigmentation at regional and national conferences should be strongly encouraged. For programs that have little exposure to skin of color, treatment of pigmentary disorders, or surgical treatment of vitiligo, externships to centers focused on these areas should be arranged. All of these methods will serve to fill current educational gaps.

CLINICAL PRACTICE AND TREATMENT GAPS

Clinical practices are largely determined by training received in residency. Most clinicians will continue to practice what they learned as a resident, with minor changes based on updates received at continuing medical education (CME) meetings, journal clubs, conferences, or through literature review. As such, many of the educational gaps formed during residency develop into practice gaps.

Melasma/Postinflammatory Hyperpigmentation

According to a study by Kang and colleagues,[1] a search of the National Ambulatory Medical Care Survey showed that the top three medications prescribed for dyschromias, including hyperpigmentation and hypopigmentation, were corticosteroids, hydroquinone, and retinoids. Photoprotection, although being the third most common treatment option in Caucasians, was sixth among African Americans and tenth among Asians. Combination therapy with hydroquinone, corticosteroid, and retinoid was prescribed less frequently in the Hispanic and African American populations, which is considered a first-line treatment for melasma and PIH along with photoprotection, even though these disorders occur more frequently in patients with skin of color.

Other gaps in clinical practice include underuse of hydroquinone alternatives in the treatment of melasma or PIH; this is especially useful because most of these agents are available over the counter at a reasonable price. Many patients are unable to afford hydroquinone combination products because they are not covered by insurance. Also, physicians who were not exposed to lasers during their residency, do not have a laser at their practice, or do not feel proficient performing chemical peels, especially in ethnic skin, will be less likely to use procedural methods.

With respect to vitiligo, one of the main practice gaps is underutilization of phototherapy, especially home phototherapy. This underutilization of home phototherapy is due to educational gaps in residency, but also because there are no definite guidelines for the prescription of phototherapy. Agents for stabilization, such as minipulse oral steroids or minocycline, are also underused, because these are more recent additions to the literature. Surgical procedures, which are performed at a minority of academic centers and practices in the United States, are effective in repigmenting vitiligo lesions in appropriate candidates. However, many physicians do not know about the efficacy or availability of surgical procedures and do not offer them as options to their patients. Physicians who want their patients evaluated for vitiligo surgery may not know to whom to refer their patients.

The solutions to clinical practice deficits are similar to those for educational practices. Clinicians first need to realize that practice gaps exist. Then, an effort needs to be made to review relevant literature. Although there are several treatment updates available on dyspigmentation, it may be difficult for physicians to know what articles are important or to make extra time for reading in the setting of busy clinical practices. These topics can be focused on during CME meetings, teleconferences, and journal clubs. Also, lectures specific to dyspigmentation should be attended at conferences. Physicians can also spend time at institutions that specialize in disorders of pigmentation to learn updated information about procedural and surgical options. With respect to vitiligo surgery, it would be helpful to have a list of institutions that perform vitiligo surgery on the AAD and American Society for Dermatologic Surgery websites. Also, in order to better guide clinical practice, experts in disorders of pigmentation should define standards of care for areas that have not been previously addressed, such as phototherapy in vitiligo. Of note, the Vitiligo Working Group is currently in the process of developing a consensus statement for the prescription of phototherapy in vitiligo. Editors and publishers should also include separate sections in their textbooks that cover these diseases and how they appear in different populations.

Given that disorders of pigmentation, specifically melasma, PIH, and vitiligo, affect such a large portion of the patient population in dermatology, it is essential that dermatologists recognize that treatment gaps exist in resident education and clinical practice. By addressing these deficits, patients will receive optimal therapy, translating into improvements in satisfaction and quality of life.

REFERENCES

1. Kang SJ, Davis SA, Feldman SR, et al. Dyschromia in skin of color. J Drugs Dermatol 2014;13(4):401–6.
2. Rossi AM, Perez MI. Treatment of hyperpigmentation. Facial Plast Surg Clin North Am 2011;19(2):313–24.
3. Molinar VE, Taylor SC, Pandya AG. What's new in objective assessment and treatment of facial hyperpigmentation? Dermatol Clin 2014;32(2):123–35.
4. Rodrigues M, Pandya AG. Melasma: clinical diagnosis and management options. Australas J Dermatol 2015;56(3):151–63.
5. Savory SA, Agim NG, Mao R, et al. Reliability assessment and validation of the postacne hyperpigmentation index (PAHPI), a new instrument to measure postinflammatory hyperpigmentation from acne vulgaris. J Am Acad Dermatol 2014;70(1):108–14.
6. Isedeh P, Kohli I, Al-Jamal M, et al. An in vivo model for postinflammatory hyperpigmentation: an analysis of histological, spectroscopic, colorimetric, and clinical traits. Br J Dermatol 2015. [Epub ahead of print].
7. Gupta AK, Gover MD, Nouri K, et al. The treatment of melasma: a review of clinical trials. J Am Acad Dermatol 2006;55(6):1048–65.
8. Liebel F, Kaur S, Ruvolo E, et al. Irradiation of skin with visible light induces reactive oxygen species and matrix-degrading enzymes. J Invest Dermatol 2012;132(7):1901–7.
9. Mahmoud BH, Ruvolo E, Hexsel CL, et al. Impact of long-wavelength UVA and visible light on melanocompetent skin. J Invest Dermatol 2010;130(8):2092–7.
10. Boukari F, Jourdan E, Fontas E, et al. Prevention of melasma relapses with sunscreen combining protection against UV and short wavelengths of visible light: a prospective randomized comparative trial. J Am Acad Dermatol 2015;72(1):189–90.e181.
11. Castanedo-Cazares JP, Hernandez-Blanco D, Carlos-Ortega B, et al. Near-visible light and UV photoprotection in the treatment of melasma: a double-blind randomized trial. Photodermatol Photoimmunol Photomed 2014;30(1):35–42.
12. Alexis AF. New and emerging treatments for hyperpigmentation. J Drugs Dermatol 2014;13(4):382–5.
13. Alexis AF, Blackcloud P. Natural ingredients for darker skin types: growing options for hyperpigmentation. J Drugs Dermatol 2013;12(9 Suppl):s123–7.
14. Dahl A, Yatskayer M, Raab S, et al. Tolerance and efficacy of a product containing ellagic and salicylic acids in reducing hyperpigmentation and dark spots in comparison with 4% hydroquinone. J Drugs Dermatol 2013;12(1):52–8.
15. Tse TW, Hui E. Tranexamic acid: an important adjuvant in the treatment of melasma. J Cosmet Dermatol 2013;12(1):57–66.
16. Nestor M, Bucay V, Callender V, et al. Polypodium leucotomos as an adjunct treatment of pigmentary disorders. J Clin Aesthet Dermatol 2014;7(3):13–7.
17. Kauvar AN. Successful treatment of melasma using a combination of microdermabrasion and Q-switched Nd:YAG lasers. Lasers Surg Med 2012;44(2):117–24.
18. Trelles MA, Velez M, Gold MH. The treatment of melasma with topical creams alone, CO2 fractional ablative resurfacing alone, or a combination of the two: a comparative study. J Drugs Dermatol 2010;9(4):315–22.
19. Daniel BS, Wittal R. Vitiligo treatment update. Australas J Dermatol 2015;56(2):85–92.
20. Laddha NC, Dwivedi M, Mansuri MS, et al. Vitiligo: interplay between oxidative stress and immune system. Exp Dermatol 2013;22(4):245–50.
21. Faria AR, Tarle RG, Dellatorre G, et al. Vitiligo–Part 2–classification, histopathology and treatment. An Bras Dermatol 2014;89(5):784–90.
22. Komen L, da Graca V, Wolkerstorfer A, et al. Vitiligo Area Scoring Index and Vitiligo European Task Force assessment: reliable and responsive instruments to measure the degree of depigmentation in vitiligo. Br J Dermatol 2015;172(2):437–43.
23. Lilly E, Lu PD, Borovicka JH, et al. Development and validation of a vitiligo-specific quality-of-life instrument (VitiQoL). J Am Acad Dermatol 2013;69(1):e11–8.
24. Gupta V, Sreenivas V, Mehta M, et al. Measurement properties of the Vitiligo Impact Scale-22 (VIS-22), a vitiligo-specific quality-of-life instrument. Br J Dermatol 2014;171(5):1084–90.
25. Taieb A, Alomar A, Bohm M, et al. Guidelines for the management of vitiligo: the European Dermatology Forum consensus. Br J Dermatol 2013;168(1):5–19.
26. Hercogova J, Buggiani G, Prignano F, et al. A rational approach to the treatment of vitiligo and

other hypomelanoses. Dermatol Clin 2007;25(3): 383–92, ix.

27. Lotti T, Buggiani G, Troiano M, et al. Targeted and combination treatments for vitiligo. Comparative evaluation of different current modalities in 458 subjects. Dermatol Ther 2008;21(Suppl 1):S20–6.

28. Majid I. Efficacy of targeted narrowband ultraviolet B therapy in vitiligo. Indian J Dermatol 2014;59(5): 485–9.

29. Falabella R. Surgical approaches for stable vitiligo. Dermatol Surg 2005;31(10):1277–84.

30. Mulekar SV, Isedeh P. Surgical interventions for vitiligo: an evidence-based review. Br J Dermatol 2013;169(Suppl 3):57–66.

31. Zhang Y, Mooneyan-Ramchurn JS, Zuo N, et al. Vitiligo nonsurgical treatment: a review of latest treatment researches. Dermatol Ther 2014;27(5): 298–303.

32. Singh A, Kanwar AJ, Parsad D, et al. Randomized controlled study to evaluate the effectiveness of dexamethasone oral minipulse therapy versus oral minocycline in patients with active vitiligo vulgaris. Indian J Dermatol Venereol Leprol 2014;80(1):29–35.

33. Whitton ME, Pinart M, Batchelor J, et al. Interventions for vitiligo. Cochrane Database Syst Rev 2015;(2):CD003263.

34. Dogra S, Kumar B. Repigmentation in vitiligo universalis: role of melanocyte density, disease duration, and melanocytic reservoir. Dermatol Online J 2005; 11(3):30.

35. Craiglow BG, King BA. Tofacitinib citrate for the treatment of vitiligo: a pathogenesis-directed therapy. JAMA Dermatol 2015;151(10):1110–2.

36. Lim HW, Grimes PE, Agbai O, et al. Afamelanotide and narrowband UV-B phototherapy for the treatment of vitiligo: a randomized multicenter trial. JAMA Dermatol 2015;151(1):42–50.

37. Anbar TS, Hegazy RA, Picardo M, et al. Beyond vitiligo guidelines: combined stratified/personalized approaches for the vitiligo patient. Exp Dermatol 2014;23(4):219–23.

38. Khunger N, Molpariya A, Khunger A. Complications of tattoos and tattoo removal: stop and think before you ink. J Cutan Aesthet Surg 2015;8(1):30–6.

39. Lotti T, Gori A, Zanieri F, et al. Vitiligo: new and emerging treatments. Dermatol Ther 2008;21(2):110–7.

40. Wolff K, Johnson RA, Saavendra AP. Pigmentary disorders. In: Wolff K, Johnson RA, Saavedra AP, editors. Fitzpatrick's color atlas and synopsis of clinical dermatology. 7th edition. New York: McGraw-Hill Education LLC; 2013. p. 284–300.

41. Chang MW. Disorders of hyperpigmentation. In: Bolognia JL, Jorizzo JL, Schaffer JV, editors. Dermatology. 3rd edition. China: Elsevier Saunders; 2012. p. 1049, 1052–4.

42. Ogden S, Griffiths C. Melasma. In: Lebwohl MG, Heymann WR, Berth-Jones J, et al, editors. Treatment of skin disease: comprehensive therapeutic strategies. 4th edition. China: Elsevier Saunders; 2014. p. 447–9.

43. Barral DC, Seabra MC, Dell'Angelica EC, et al. Disturbances of pigmentation. In: James WD, Berger TG, Elston DM, editors. Andrews' diseases of the skin clinical dermatology. 11th edition. London: Elsevier Saunders; 2011. p. 847–8, 854–857.

44. The 2014/2015 Derm in-review study guide. Educational Testing and Assessment Systems; 2014.

45. Harris JE, Picardo M, Henderson M, et al. Annual meeting program book. San Diego: Paper Presented at American Academy of Dermatology; 2015. March 20-24.

46. Ortonne JP, Passeron T. Vitiligo and other disorders of hypopigmentation. In: Bolognia JL, Jorizzo JL, Schaffer JV, editors. Dermatology. 3rd edition. China: Elsevier Saunders; 2012. p. 1023–37.

47. Lebwohl MG, Heymann WR, Berth-Jones J, et al, editors. Treatment of skin disease: comprehensive therapeutic strategies. 4th edition. China: Elsevier Saunders; 2014. p. 794–8.

48. Nijhawan RI, Jacob SE, Woolery-Lloyd H. Skin of color education in dermatology residency programs: does residency training reflect the changing demographics of the United States? J Am Acad Dermatol 2008;59(4):615–8.

49. Tien Guan ST, Theng C, Chang A. Randomized, parallel group trial comparing home-based phototherapy with institution-based 308 excimer lamp for the treatment of focal vitiligo vulgaris. J Am Acad Dermatol 2015;72(4):733–5.

50. Wind BS, Kroon MW, Beek JF, et al. Home vs. outpatient narrowband ultraviolet B therapy for the treatment of nonsegmental vitiligo: a retrospective questionnaire study. Br J Dermatol 2010;162(5): 1142–4.

51. Anderson KL, Huang KE, Huang WW, et al. Dermatology resident training and comfort in prescribing in-office and home phototherapy. Paper Presented at 24th Annual Meeting of The Photomedicine Society. March 19, San Francisco, CA, 2015.

52. Fisk WA, Agbai O, Lev-Tov HA, et al. The use of botanically derived agents for hyperpigmentation: a systematic review. J Am Acad Dermatol 2014; 70(2):352–65.

53. Fowler JF Jr, Woolery-Lloyd H, Waldorf H, et al. Innovations in natural ingredients and their use in skin care. J Drugs Dermatol 2010;9(6 Suppl):S72–81 [quiz: S82–3].

54. Panich U, Kongtaphan K, Onkoksoong T, et al. Modulation of antioxidant defense by Alpinia galanga and Curcuma aromatica extracts correlates with their inhibition of UVA-induced melanogenesis. Cell Biol Toxicol 2010;26(2):103–16.

55. Konda S, Geria AN, Halder RM. New horizons in treating disorders of hyperpigmentation in skin of color. Semin Cutan Med Surg 2012;31(2):133–9.

Practice and Educational Gaps in Genodermatoses

Julie V. Schaffer, MD

KEYWORDS

- Genodermatoses • Genetic counseling • Genetic testing • Next-generation sequencing
- Phenotype

KEY POINTS

- The recent explosion in genetic knowledge has not yet been fully incorporated into clinical dermatology practice or dermatology resident education.
- The interface between dermatology and genetics has expanded with recognition of new heritable disorders and broader phenotypic spectrums; updated classification systems integrate clinical and molecular data, clarifying relationships among conditions.
- Online databases and next-generation sequencing provide important tools for the diagnosis of genodermatoses.
- This article highlights strategies to overcome barriers and correct practice and educational gaps, enhancing the ability of dermatologists to diagnose, counsel, evaluate, and treat patients and families affected by genodermatoses.

INTRODUCTION

In recent years, there has been tremendous progress in determining the molecular bases of genodermatoses,[1,2] with greater than 1000 genes now associated with a cutaneous phenotype. A paradigm shift is occurring in genetic skin disease, with revised definitions and classification of these conditions and considerable expansion of their limits. Genodermatoses are no longer confined to a small group of rare, clearly familial, monogenic disorders that become apparent by early childhood. It is important that dermatologists be aware of the spectrum of clinical presentations of genetic skin disease in patients of all ages as well as the many recent advances in available diagnostic studies and (for some conditions) molecularly directed treatments.

GENODERMATOSES IN CLINICAL DERMATOLOGY PRACTICE
Characterization and Classification of Patients with Genodermatoses

Begin with the basics
When evaluating patients suspected to have genodermatosis, the first step is a thorough history and review of systems, together with a complete dermatologic examination that includes the hair, nails, oral mucosa, and teeth. Results of previous histologic, radiographic, and laboratory studies should be collected. To help establish the mode of inheritance, history and (if applicable) physical examination should be used to determine whether or not family members have similar findings.

Gaps in current practice The short time allotted for most dermatology visits makes it difficult to fully

The author has nothing to disclose.
Division of Pediatric Dermatology, Hackensack University Medical Center, 155 Polifly Road, Suite 101, Hackensack, NJ 07601, USA
E-mail address: jschaffer@hackensackumc.org

Dermatol Clin 34 (2016) 303–310
http://dx.doi.org/10.1016/j.det.2016.02.007
0733-8635/16/$ – see front matter © 2016 Elsevier Inc. All rights reserved.

assess patients with complicated histories and multisystem findings. Logistical problems getting access to previous records may lead to unnecessary and costly repetition of testing. Potentially affected family members may be deceased, live far away, or not be available for assessment; and descriptions may be inaccurate. Furthermore, assessment of complex disease and recognition of patterns of inheritance can be challenging and outside the comfort zone of general dermatologists.

Strategies to overcome barriers Longer or additional visits would ideally be planned for patients with complex or multisystem disease. Appropriate release forms should be obtained to enable access to medical records. Assessment of family members may require review of photographs or collaboration with dermatologists and other physicians in their region.

Genetic skin disease clinics providing specialized multidisciplinary care that includes genetics as well as dermatology services are becoming more widely available with the expansion of pediatric dermatology centers, but more are needed. Involving patients' primary physicians can be helpful, and referrals to geneticists and other subspecialists should be made as indicated.

Clinical characterization and classification
It is useful to first categorize patients with genodermatoses based on the general type of primary skin finding.[1,3] Examples include, mechanical fragility/blister formation, abnormal cornification, hypopigmentation or hyperpigmentation, adnexal anomalies (eg, hypotrichosis, ectodermal dysplasia), connective tissue or vascular defects, and tumor predisposition.[4–8] Considering the large number of potential diagnoses and genetic causes within each category, online databases, such as Online Mendelian Inheritance in Man (OMIM) and PubMed, represent important tools.[2,9] The differential diagnosis can be narrowed based on specific clinical features, histologic findings, distribution patterns, and time courses of cutaneous manifestations as well as by the presence or absence of associated extracutaneous manifestations. This assessment process often helps to direct additional studies and referrals.

Gaps in current practice Unfortunately, the recent explosion in genetic knowledge has not yet been widely incorporated into clinical practice[1] (**Table 1**). The enormous amount of available information may be difficult to access, interpret, synthesize, and apply in a way that is meaningful to patient care. Although basic OMIM and PubMed have open access, individual articles may be costly to dermatologists who are not part of a university or hospital system. Moreover, navigation to obtain relevant information can be a challenge, and databases such as OMIM are not set up to provide the explicit details on cutaneous manifestations that are often required for the clinical diagnosis of genodermatoses.[1] The literature is laden with outdated and inconsistent terminology using descriptive names, eponyms, and synonyms. Multiple complex and disparate classification systems also add to the confusion and potential for misdiagnosis.[10]

As a result of the tremendous progress in elucidating the genetic bases of inherited skin disorders, the large number of genetically distinct conditions in categories such as epidermolysis bullosa (EB), ichthyoses, and ectodermal dysplasias can be overwhelming.[4,5,8] The phenotypic spectrum of a particular disorder often extends beyond the classic textbook presentation, with milder, late-onset, atypical, or mosaic variants. Infants and young children may have incomplete or nonspecific phenotypes before the development of key diagnostic features, whereas conditions with delayed onset may not be recognized as genetic in origin. In addition, as many new genetic skin diseases have been identified, the limits of genodermatoses have been expanded to include entities previously considered as acquired, including predisposition to particular infections and inflammatory disorders ranging from pustular psoriasis to interferonopathies.[11]

Clinical and genetic (locus) heterogeneity are also common and further complicate classification. *Clinical heterogeneity* in genetic diseases refers to mutations in a single gene causing more than one disorder. This clinical variability classically reflects different mutations (*allelic heterogeneity*), such as *TP63* mutations that affect various domains of the p63 protein leading to separate types of ectodermal dysplasia. However, clinical heterogeneity sometimes results from the same mutation occurring in patients with other genetic differences. For example, identical germline mutations in the *PTEN* gene can result in early onset Bannayan-Riley-Ruvalcaba syndrome versus later-onset Cowden syndrome, depending on the timing and extent of somatic second-hit *PTEN* mutations. Conversely, *genetic heterogeneity* refers to mutations in different genes producing the same clinical disorder, which often occurs when the encoded proteins interact with one another in a complex or signaling pathway.[10]

Strategies to overcome barriers Attempts are being made to integrate molecular and clinical data in order to simplify genodermatosis classification, better define disease spectrums, and eliminate

Table 1
Summary of clinical practice gaps for genodermatoses

Goal	Best Practice Strategies	Barriers to Best Practice Implementation	Strategies to Overcome Barriers
Disease characterization and classification	• Thorough personal and family history, review of systems, dermatologic examination, and evaluation of the medical record • Categorize based on primary skin findings • Consider alternative diagnostic possibilities • Use online databases (eg, OMIM, PubMed) to narrow the DDx based on additional features and to plan further evaluation	• Limited time and resources • Patients often previously misdiagnosed • Huge numbers of genetic conditions and genes • Difficulties in accessing, interpreting, synthesizing, and applying information • Confusing classification systems and terminology • Ill-defined, broad phenotypic spectrums with clinical and genetic heterogeneity	• Plan longer/additional visits • Keep an open mind to other diagnostic possibilities • Seek input from experts/specialists and support groups • Use accessible resources (eg, GeneReviews) • Use updated classification systems that integrate clinical and molecular data, better define phenotypic spectrums, and clarify relationships among conditions
Molecular diagnosis	• Recognize the options available for genetic testing • Find a laboratory that performs the desired testing (eg, via www.genetests.org) • Determine the rationale for testing and provide counseling to patients/families	• Lack of awareness of newer genetic testing options, available laboratory services, costs, diagnostic implications, or limitations • Little experience counseling patients and families about relevant issues • Inadequate insurance coverage/prohibitive costs	• Use online directories • Seek input from geneticists/genetic counselors • Consider research laboratory-based testing if clinical testing is not possible
Management	• Symptomatic treatment • Avoidance or early detection of complications • Patient/family education • Multidisciplinary care as indicated	• Little experience with rare conditions • Patients/families feel isolated and frustrated that no magic bullet of gene therapy is available	• Refer to disease-specific multidisciplinary clinics • Seek input from experts/specialists and support groups • Ongoing investigations of gene-, cell-, and protein-based therapies as well as treatments targeting the affected molecular pathway

Abbreviation: DDx, differential diagnosis.

redundant terminology. This process has been successfully accomplished for disorders, such as EB and ichthyoses; however, it represents a work in progress, to be continually refined as additional genotype-phenotype correlations are established.[4,5] In addition, grouping hereditary skin disorders according to their molecular bases highlights relationships between conditions and their shared pathomechanisms (see later discussion).

Once a patient's condition is categorized, further user-friendly information and assistance can be obtained from accessible online resources, such as expert-authored GeneReview summaries and support groups, with examples including the Dystrophic EB Research Association (DEBRA; www.debra.org or www.debra-international.org), Foundation for Ichthyosis and Related Skin Types (FIRST; www.firstskinfoundation.org), and National Foundation for Ectodermal Dysplasias (www.nfed.org). Other options include referral to genetic skin disease or other specialty clinics and potentially obtaining expert consultation via teledermatology.

Keep an open mind to alternative diagnoses
Because most genodermatoses are rare and there is little awareness of these disorders among the medical community, patients often present with another "established" diagnosis. It is important that dermatologists consider alternative possibilities that may have a better fit and make referrals to specialists as indicated.

Gaps in current practice In a recent survey, patients with rare diseases in the United Kingdom and United States reported an average delay of 5 to 8 years before their diagnosis was determined. During this time, they saw an average of 8 physicians and received 2 to 3 incorrect diagnoses,[12] which often led to costly investigations and inappropriate treatments.

Strategies to overcome barriers Take a fresh look at patients without preexisting labels, and do not be afraid to expand the differential diagnosis.

Molecular Diagnosis in Patients with Genodermatoses

Recognize available options for genetic testing
Detection of a germline (constitutional) mutation can be accomplished via analysis of DNA from a blood sample (1–5 mL in ethylenediaminetetraacetic acid) or oral rinse/buccal brush specimen (which may not be adequate for some tests). For type 1 mosaic conditions, which are caused by a dominant heterozygous postzygotic mutation, identification of the underlying mutation often

requires DNA to be obtained from a sample of affected tissue. In contrast, a mutation can be detected in a standard blood or oral/buccal sample from patients with type 2 mosaic conditions, which are due to a postzygotic second hit in the setting of a heterozygous germline mutation, as well as in female patients with X-linked genodermatoses who present with skin lesions along Blaschko lines due to functional mosaicism.

Traditional genetic testing involves analysis of the genes that cause a particular disorder through bidirectional sequencing (Sanger method). This method may be used in conjunction with mutation scanning to identify variant regions, deletion/duplication analysis, and other methods, such as RNA studies to assess for splice site mutations in introns. The turnaround time for assessment of a single gene is typically in the range of 2 to 10 weeks. When a condition is often caused by certain hot-spot mutations, a tiered approach first targeting these mutations or sequencing selected high-yield exons can be used. Sequencing particular exons first may also be recommended for patients with phenotypic features or ethnic backgrounds associated with specific mutations.

Multigene panels enable a large group of genes associated with a particular phenotype to be evaluated in a cost-effective manner.[13,14] These tests use next-generation sequencing, a rapid process in which millions of small DNA segments are analyzed at the same time.[15] Multigene panels are especially valuable for conditions and phenotypes that have substantial genetic heterogeneity. Currently available multigene panels that may be useful to dermatologists include those for EB, ichthyoses, albinism, RASopathies, and periodic fever syndromes. Customized panels targeting genes associated with phenotypes and molecular pathways relevant to an individual patient can also be designed.

Whole-exome sequencing (WES) and *whole-genome sequencing* (WGS) represent important tools in gene discovery and are options in patients with a constellation of clinical manifestations that are not typical of a disorder with a known genetic basis.[16,17] WES and WGS are offered by a growing number of university-based medical centers and companies. In addition, the National Institutes of Health Centers for Mendelian Genomics work with collaborating investigators to provide WES/WGS and extensive analysis for patients with Mendelian phenotypes with unknown genetic causes.[18,19]

Gaps in current practice Practicing dermatologists may not be aware of the possible applications of traditional genetic testing or newer next-generation sequencing approaches for diagnosis of genodermatoses. For example, panels that include all known EB genes can potentially serve as a sensitive primary diagnostic test for this group of conditions, with increased availability and decreased costs likely in the future.[14,20,21]

Although the potential of WES/WGS is exciting, its overall success rate in finding the causative gene for Mendelian disorders is currently only approximately 20% to 50%.[22] Further filtering of the genomic deluge of data requires computational tools that use published reference sequences, predicted effects on protein function, and phenotypic information.[23,24]

Strategies to overcome barriers Dermatology textbooks, review articles, and educational meetings need to provide dermatologists with updated, practical information on the genetic testing methods available for patients with genodermatoses (**Table 2**). Dermatologists should work

together with geneticists and genetic counselors in determining the best approach for individual patients and families.

The yield of WES/WGS is increased by analysis of a trio including patients and both biological parents.[22] The challenge is not in finding genetic variants but rather in determining which variant is responsible for the disease. Methods of processing the huge amounts of data generated by WES/WGS are still being optimized.[23,24] Because larger sample sizes are required to prove causality for mutations in new genes, collaborative efforts using networking and online databases will be crucial.[10]

Find a laboratory for genetic testing
When molecular testing is desired for a suspected condition or group of conditions with a known genetic basis, it is important to determine what options are available in clinical laboratories. The GeneTests (www.genetests.org) and Genetic

---

Table 2
Summary of educational gaps for genodermatoses

Component of Dermatology Resident Education	Best Educational Approach	Barriers to Best Approach Implementation	Strategies to Overcome Barriers
Basic science curriculum on genodermatoses	• Emphasize conceptual understanding of the molecular structures and pathways that are disrupted • Learn to use online databases (eg, OMIM, PubMed) to access, interpret, and synthesize genetic information • Recognize patterns of inheritance, forms of mosaicism, genotype-phenotype correlations, and methods of disease gene identification	• Dermatology residents traditionally memorize increasingly long lists of the genes that cause various skin diseases.	• Focus teaching and examination preparation on the relevance of genes and related molecular pathways to mechanisms of disease, therapeutic decisions, and diagnostic tests • Use molecular classification to highlight relationships between conditions and shared pathomechanisms
Clinical curriculum on genodermatoses	• Emphasize the spectrum of clinical features, natural history, evaluation, and management • Gain experience counseling and educating patients/families	• Dermatology residents may have little or no clinical exposure to some rare conditions.	• Use encounters with patients with genodermatoses as opportunities to teach/learn about the DDx and other conditions in that category • Enhance exposure via case presentations and educational sessions with patient viewing

Abbreviation: DDx, differential diagnosis.

Testing Registry (www.ncbi.nlm.nih.gov/gtr/) websites provide up-to-date directories of international clinical genetic laboratories that can be searched by gene symbol, affected protein, or disease name.

Although new technologies have led to some decreases in costs, genetic analysis remains expensive. It is crucial to ascertain and discuss with patients/families the price of the test, coverage by the patients' insurance, other payment options (eg, institutional billing, self-pay), and the projected out-of-pocket cost. If clinical testing is not possible, a scientist who studies that gene in a research laboratory may be willing to perform the analysis on an investigational basis; research results that are released to patients should be confirmed in a certified clinical laboratory.

Gaps in current practice Dermatologists may not be aware of resources to determine the laboratory services available for genetic testing or the potential costs involved. In some instances, insurance coverage is inadequate and the costs are prohibitive.[25]

Strategies to overcome barriers Provide dermatologists with information on online directories of genetic testing options. Encourage collaboration with geneticists and genetic counselors who can help facilitate the process.

Determine the rationale for testing and provide counseling

Before performing genetic analysis in patients suspected to have a genodermatosis, the potential benefits, limitations, and risks should be carefully considered and discussed with the affected individuals and/or families. Confirmation of the diagnosis could affect patients' prognosis, monitoring, and treatment.[26,27] Additional implications include the ability to diagnose asymptomatic family members at risk of the condition (eg, those younger than the usual age of clinical onset), determine whether family members are carriers, and perform prenatal/preimplantation genetic diagnosis. In some situations whereby the diagnosis can be established by other means, genetic testing may not provide further benefit. An example would be a young child with an autosomal recessive form of EB diagnosed by immunofluorescence mapping whose parents do not plan to have more children.

Counseling for patients and families receiving genetic testing should include an explanation of basic genetic terms (eg, gene, mutation), inheritance patterns, and concepts such as penetrance and variable expressivity. The possibility of detecting gene variants that are neutral or have an unknown effect as well as pathogenic/disease-causing mutations should be reviewed.[28] Mutation-detection rates vary among patients meeting clinical diagnostic criteria for various genodermatoses, ranging from greater than 95% to less than 60%. Potential explanations for false-negative findings include genetic alterations not detectable by the methods used, mosaicism, genetic heterogeneity (see earlier discussion), and laboratory error; false-positive results are also possible.

Other relevant issues may include confidentiality and (if parental samples are obtained) potential detection of nonpaternity. For WES/WGS, a plan for possible incidental findings in a gene unrelated to the disease being investigated should be addressed. This plan may depend on whether the finding is medically actionable and the projected age of clinical onset. In the United States, the Genetic Information Nondiscrimination Act of 2008 provides protection in health insurance and employment settings; however, it does not include all possible forms of genetic discrimination (eg, life or disability insurance). Many state governments require documentation of consent for performance of genetic testing and disclosure of genetic information.

Gaps in current practice Dermatologists may not be aware of the diagnostic implications and limitations of genetic testing. Furthermore, they may have little experience counseling patients about inheritance patterns and other issues relevant to genetic testing.

Strategies to overcome barriers Provide dermatologists with information on genetic testing and encourage referral of patients/families affected by genodermatoses for genetic counseling. Genetic counselors can help to educate patients and families about genetic testing and the potential implications for family members. They also provide psychological support and assist in family planning.

Management of Patients with Genodermatoses

Management of patients with genodermatoses primarily involves symptomatic treatment and avoidance or early detection of complications, which often require the input of other specialists. Counseling about the expected natural history, inheritance pattern, and issues related to family planning are critical components of care.

Gaps in current practice

Patients and families affected by genodermatoses may feel isolated, and the dermatologists caring for them may have little experience in managing these rare conditions. The accessibility of the skin makes it an excellent target for gene therapy, but the routine application of this treatment modality is not currently possible.

Strategies to overcome barriers

As noted earlier, multidisciplinary clinics devoted to genetic skin disease or a particular subgroup, such as EB, can be of great benefit; teledermatology may potentially be used to obtain expert consultation. Patients, families, and physicians can also obtain helpful information and support from disease-specific organizations/websites such as DEBRA and FIRST (see earlier discussion).

Steps have been taken to study the feasibility of gene therapy for heritable skin diseases, especially in patients with EB.[29] Cell- and protein-based therapies for EB and other conditions, such as hypohidrotic ectodermal dysplasia, are also under investigation. Understanding the molecular pathway that is affected in a group of genodermatoses can translate into effective therapy, with examples ranging from mammalian target of rapamycin inhibitors for tuberous sclerosis and *PTEN* hamartoma tumor syndrome to topical cholesterol and lovastatin in congenital hemidysplasia with ichthyosis and limb defects syndrome.[30]

GENODERMATOSES IN DERMATOLOGY RESIDENT EDUCATION
Basic Science Curriculum on Genodermatoses

With the recent flood of genetic information, dermatologists are not expected to know all of the greater than 1000 genes involved in skin disease, although they should know how to access this information through up-to-date online resources (eg, OMIM, PubMed). Instead, dermatology resident education should emphasize conceptual understanding of the key molecular structures and pathways that are disrupted in patients with genodermatoses. This understanding frequently provides insights into cutaneous physiology and the pathogenesis of more common multifactorial disorders. Additional topics related to the genetics of cutaneous disease that should be covered include Mendelian patterns of inheritance and modifying factors, forms of mosaicism due to genetic changes and X-inactivation, genotype-phenotype correlations, and methods of disease gene identification.

Gaps in current dermatology education

Dermatology residents often spend time memorizing long lists of the genes that cause various skin diseases. This practice does not provide meaningful insights into mechanisms of disease and is not a focus of current American Board of Dermatology examinations.

Strategies to overcome barriers

Dermatology resident education and examination preparation should focus on the relevance of genes and related molecular pathways to mechanisms of skin disease, therapeutic decisions, and diagnostic tests. Considering the huge number of genes implicated in skin disease, molecular classification represents a useful approach that highlights relationships between conditions, their shared pathomechanisms, and potential therapeutic targets.[11,30,31] For example, it explains the overlapping clinical features of the various RASopathies that activate the RAS/mitogen-activated protein kinase pathway and gives insights into the lipid metabolism defects that link classic ichthyoses with metabolic disorders, such as Gaucher disease (which can also present with ichthyosiform skin).[31]

Clinical Curriculum on Genodermatoses

Dermatology residents should learn the spectrum of clinical presentations of genetic skin diseases, associated extracutaneous manifestations, pertinent histopathologic findings, and the expected time course. Their training should include appropriate radiographic and laboratory investigations to diagnose and manage patients with inherited skin disorders and awareness of emerging therapeutic options. Residents should also gain experience in educating and counseling patients and families affected by genodermatoses.

Gaps in current dermatology education

Because many genodermatoses are rare, dermatology residents may have little or no clinical exposure to some conditions during their training.

Strategies to overcome barriers

Although individually rare, as a whole, the group of genodermatoses is relatively common,[32] especially when expanded to include mosaic disorders, such as epidermal and congenital melanocytic nevi. Encounters with patients with genodermatosis can be used as opportunities to teach and learn about the differential diagnosis as well as other conditions in that category, for example, ichthyoses, types of EB, and disorders presenting with multiple café-au-lait macules. Case presentations and educational sessions with patient viewing represent additional opportunities for exposure to rare diseases.

REFERENCES

1. Lemke JR, Kernland-Lang K, Hörtnagel K, et al. Monogenic human skin disorders. Dermatology 2014;229:55–64.

2. Feramisco JD, Sadreyev RI, Murray ML, et al. Phenotypic and genotypic analyses of genetic skin disease through the Online Mendelian Inheritance in Man (OMIM) database. J Invest Dermatol 2009; 129:2628–36.

3. Feramisco JD, Tsao H, Siegel DH. Genetics for the practicing dermatologist. Semin Cutan Med Surg 2010;29:127–36.

4. Oji V, Tadini G, Akiyama M, et al. Revised nomenclature and classification of inherited ichthyoses: results of the First Ichthyosis Consensus Conference in Sorèze 2009. J Am Acad Dermatol 2010;63:607–41.

5. Fine J-D, Bruckner-Tuderman L, Eady RAJ, et al. Inherited epidermolysis bullosa (EB): updated recommendations on diagnosis and classification. J Am Acad Dermatol 2014;70:1103–26.

6. Betz RC, Cabral RM, Christiano AM, et al. Unveiling the roots of monogenic genodermatoses: genotrichoses as a paradigm. J Invest Dermatol 2012; 132:906–14.

7. Ponti G, Pellacani G, Seidenari S, et al. Cancer-associated genodermatoses: skin neoplasms as clues to hereditary tumor syndromes. Crit Rev Oncol Hematol 2013;85:239–56.

8. Pagnan NA, Visinoni AF. Update on ectodermal dysplasias clinical classification. Am J Med Genet A 2014;164A:2415–23.

9. McKusick VA. Mendelian inheritance in man and its online version, OMIM. Am J Hum Genet 2007;80: 588–604.

10. Schaffer JV. Molecular diagnostics in genodermatoses. Semin Cutan Med Surg 2012;31:211–20.

11. Crow YJ, Manel N. Aicardi-Goutières syndrome and the type I interferonopathies. Nat Rev Immunol 2015; 15:429–40.

12. Rare disease impact report: insights from patients and the medical community. GlobalGenes.org/wp-content/uploads/2013/04/ShireReport-1.pdf. Accessed June 17, 2016.

13. Klee EW, Hoppman-Chaney NL, Ferber MJ. Expanding DNA diagnostic panel testing: is more better? Expert Rev Mol Diagn 2011;11:703–9.

14. Cho RJ, Simpson MA, McGrath JA. Next-generation diagnostics for genodermatoses. J Invest Dermatol 2012;132:E27–8.

15. Metzker M. Sequencing technologies – the next generation. Nat Rev Genet 2010;11:31–46.

16. Bamshad MJ, Ng SB, Bigham AW, et al. Exome sequencing as a tool for Mendelian disease gene discovery. Nat Rev Genet 2011;12:745–55.

17. Precone V, Del Monaco V, Esposito MV, et al. Cracking the code of human diseases using next-generation sequencing: applications, challenges, and perspectives. Biomed Res Int 2015;2015: 161648.

18. Bamshad MJ, Shendure JA, Valle D, et al. The centers for Mendelian genomics: a new large-scale initiative to identify the genes underlying rare Mendelian conditions. Am J Med Genet A 2012;158A: 1523–5.

19. Chong JX, Buckingham KJ, Jhangiani SN, et al. The genetic basis of Mendelian phenotypes: discoveries, challenges, and opportunities. Am J Hum Genet 2015;97:199–215.

20. Takeichi T, Liu L, Fong K, et al. Whole-exome sequencing improves mutation detection in a diagnostic epidermolysis bullosa laboratory. Br J Dermatol 2015;172:94–100.

21. Tenedini E, Artuso L, Bernardis I, et al. Amplicon-based NGS: an effective approach for the molecular diagnosis of epidermolysis bullosa. Br J Dermatol 2015;173:731–8.

22. Retterer K, Juusola J, Cho MT, et al. Clinical application of whole-exome sequencing across clinical indications. Genet Med 2015. [Epub ahead of print].

23. Javed A, Agrawal S, Ng PC. Phen-Gen: combining phenotype and genotype to analyze rare disorders. Nat Methods 2014;11:935–7.

24. Yang H, Robinson PN, Wang K. Phenolyzer: phenotype-based prioritization of candidate genes for human diseases. Nat Methods 2015;12:841–3.

25. Pandhi D. Current status of genodermatoses: an Indian perspective. Indian J Dermatol Venereol Leprol 2015;81:7–9.

26. Has C, He Y. Practical aspects of molecular diagnostics in genodermatoses. Hautarzt 2016;67(1): 53–8 [in German].

27. Laimer M, Bauer JW, Lang R. Molecular diagnostics in genodermatoses. Hautarzt 2015;66:203–11 [in German].

28. Richards S, Aziz N, Bale S, et al. Standards and guidelines for the interpretation of sequence variants: a joint consensus recommendation of the American College of Medical Genetics and Genomics and the Association for Molecular Pathology. Genet Med 2015;17:405–24.

29. Hsu CK, Wang SP, Lee JY, et al. Treatment of hereditary epidermolysis bullosa: updates and future prospects. Am J Clin Dermatol 2014;15:1–6.

30. Vahidnezhad H, Youssefian L, Uitto J. Molecular genetics of the PI3K-AKT-mTOR pathway in genodermatoses: diagnostic implications and treatment opportunities. J Invest Dermatol 2015. [Epub ahead of print].

31. Rauen KA. The RASopathies. Annu Rev Genomics Hum Genet 2013;14:355–69.

32. Itin P, Salgado DA. Important genodermatoses for the practitioner. Hautarzt 2013;64:26–31 [in German].

Practice Gaps: Drug Reactions

Stephen E. Wolverton, MD

KEYWORDS

- Drug reactions • Practice gaps • Cutaneous drug reactions • Systemic drugs

KEY POINTS

- The common categories of drug reactions include purely cutaneous drug reactions, cutaneous drug reactions with systemic features, and dermatologic systemic drugs with systemic adverse effects.
- Continuation of or rechallenge with the drug/drugs in question is generally unwise for the latter two categories.
- The Kramer algorithm from 1979 with FDA modifications has the best diagnostic certainty for drug reactions.
- The decision triad consists of literature experience, personal experience, and biologic plausibility and is a practical system for making medical decisions, including drug reaction diagnosis.
- FDA warnings or boxed warnings (black box warnings) do not require establishment of causation before publication.

INTRODUCTION

The term "drug reactions" is relevant to dermatology in three categories of reactions: (1) cutaneous drug reactions without systemic features, (2) cutaneous drug reactions with systemic features, and (3) systemic drugs prescribed by a dermatologist with systematic adverse effects. This article is not intended to be comprehensive, but instead uses three examples from each of these categories to illustrate several important principles central to drug reaction diagnosis and management. There are several important areas of overall drug safety that are not included in this article, including drug interactions and medical-legal risk management.

CATEGORIES OF DRUG REACTIONS DISCUSSED

Purely cutaneous drug reactions (Table 1) include morbilliform reactions (synonyms include exanthematous and maculopapular reactions),[1] fixed drug eruption,[2,3] and linear IgA bullous dermatosis.[4,5]

Cutaneous drug reactions with systemic features include Stevens-Johnson syndrome (SJS)/ toxic epidermal necrolysis (TEN) spectrum,[6,7] drug-induced hypersensitivity syndrome also known as drug reaction with eosinophils and systemic symptoms (DRESS),[8,9] and acute generalized exanthematous pustulosis.[10,11]

Dermatologic systemic drugs with systemic adverse effects include methotrexate (MTX)-induced chronic liver disease,[12] cyclosporine-induced chronic kidney injury,[13] and biologic therapy–induced hepatitis B reactivation.[14,15]

GENERAL PRINCIPLES

In general, clinicians work with less than 100% certainty in making most medical decisions. I have found the following decision triad to have significant clinical value in reaching the highest level of certainty possible (Table 2).

- Literature experience: with all the pitfalls discussed next, realizing there is no subject for which all articles agree
- Personal experience: direct (clinician's own experience) and indirect (shared experience of mentors and colleagues)

Department of Dermatology, Indiana University, 545 Barnhill Drive, Emerson Hall 139, Indianapolis, IN 46202, USA
E-mail address: swolvert@iu.edu

Dermatol Clin 34 (2016) 311–318
http://dx.doi.org/10.1016/j.det.2016.02.009
0733-8635/16/$ – see front matter © 2016 Elsevier Inc. All rights reserved.

Table 1
Common drug reaction by category

Purely Cutaneous Drug Reactions	Cutaneous Drug Reactions with Systemic Features	Systemic Drugs Prescribed by Dermatology with Systemic AE
Morbilliform reactions	SJS/TEN spectrum	MTX-induced chronic liver disease
Fixed drug eruptions	Drug-induced hypersensitivity syndrome/DRESS syndrome	Cyclosporine A–induced chronic kidney injury
Linear IgA bullous dermatosis	Acute generalized exanthematous pustulosis	Biologic therapy–induced hepatitis B reactivation

Abbreviations: AE, adverse events; DRESS, drug-induced hypersensitivity syndrome versus drug reaction with eosinophils and systemic symptoms; MTX, methotrexate; SJS, Stevens-Johnson syndrome; TEN, toxic epidermal necrolysis.

- Biologic plausibility: mechanistically what is logical or makes sense

There are several general limits of this decision triad. In most clinical scenarios, diagnostic level of certainty falls well short of 100% (**Table 3**). For example, in clinical trials, a significant $P = .05$ still leaves 5% possibility that the findings were caused by chance alone. Smaller P values (≤ 0.01) substantially improve the level of certainty. That example is substantially more precise than diagnosing a drug reaction in an individual patient. In general, clinicians make drug reaction diagnostic decisions using the preponderance of evidence that is available at the time the decision must be made.

A second general concept when facing a clinical decision involving a possible drug reaction is the risk/benefit ratio, where the risk of possible drug reaction is compared with the potential benefit of continuing the drug/drugs in question. Given that most of the time this clinical scenario occurs in an outpatient office setting, at least briefly discontinuing the drug/drugs in question is wise until further diagnostic evidence becomes available. A noteworthy exception to this general rule is with prednisone (or other forms of systemic corticosteroid) therapy in which abrupt cessation of therapy has significant potential risks including an addisonian crisis. However, such corticosteroid therapy is seldom central to the diagnostic decisions of any drug reactions.

PITFALLS AND LIMITATIONS IN GENERAL

Before looking closely at the proposed causation algorithm, a discussion of some general pitfalls of medical decision making concerning drug reactions is presented next. The following are no doubt influenced by the clinician's temperament and his or her inherent level of awareness for information inherent to medical decision making involving drug reaction diagnosis.

There are two types of general errors: errors of underconcern and errors of overconcern. The errors of underconcern include (1) failure to monitor for liver toxicity with dapsone and azathioprine,[16] (2) failure to screen for possible hepatitis B reactivation with biologic therapeutics for psoriasis, and (3) minimal to no MTX surveillance in an individual with multiple predictors of nonalcoholic steatohepatitis.[12] Errors of overconcern are excessive concern for a morbilliform reaction in a patient not receiving drugs known to induce DRESS syndrome; or managing morbilliform drug reactions without systemic findings of DRESS syndrome, such as the absence of eosinophilia, liver transaminase changes, or findings of acute kidney injury (urinalysis changes or rise in creatinine).[8,9] The ideal level of concern is difficult to define, but includes appropriately cautious measures to monitor for drug reactions discussed in this review.

In addition, there are two other distinct general errors clinicians commonly make. The first is failure to adapt to compelling new literature

Table 2
Decision triad

Decision Factor	Comments
Literature experience	No subject for which all articles agree
Personal experience (direct and indirect)	Generally inadequate volume of cases for statistical significance
Biologic plausibility	Mechanistically what is logical or makes sense

information (complete skepticism); this is in essence saying "don't confuse me with the facts, my mind is made up." The second is no careful analysis or scrutiny for any new literature information (complete gullibility); an example of this approach includes "the last article is always right," believing the last article published automatically negates the validity all prior articles on the same topic. A happy medium to sort out literature trends is finding a healthy skepticism. Tools for sorting out such trends are detailed in later sections.

CAUSATION DETERMINATION THROUGH AN ALGORITHM

Even with careful use of the following algorithm, diagnostic certainty typically falls well short of 100% (See **Table 3**). This is the reality all clinicians face, yet once again the preponderance of evidence needs to be used in the necessary clinical decisions; making no decision (while awaiting possible future definitive studies) generally is not a viable option. The basic algorithm[17,18] with some adaptation of the original terminology to simplify phraseology, is as follows

- *Challenge*: this is a retrospective component assessing the composite of (1) literature reputation of the drug/drugs involved in causing the specific drug reaction, (2) the clinician's personal experience both direct and indirect (as previously defined), (3) the individual patient's prior experience with the drug/drugs involved, and (4) duration the patient has taken the drug/drugs in question.
- *Dechallenge*: this is a prospective step concerning what happens to the clinical presentation of the drug reaction when the drug/drugs in question are stopped.
- *Rechallenge*: this prospective step is the most definitive step of the algorithm concerning clinical response after the drug/drugs in question are restarted (see limitations below in particular with this step)

Table 3
Causation algorithm components

Components	Subcomponents	Pitfalls
Kramer Criteria Algorithm		
Challenge	1. Literature reputation of suspected drug 2. Clinician's personal experience 3. Patient experience with drug/drugs of concern 4. Duration patient has been taking the drug in question	1. Literature reputation of drug may be unclear 2. Delayed timing from initiation of drug therapy
Dechallenge	1. Clinical response of drug reaction after drug cessation 2. Keep drug metabolism half-life in mind	1. May be partial or no resolution 2. Inherent disease activity may complicate decision making 3. Prolonged half-life in serum or fat
Rechallenge	1. Clinical response to restarting drug/drugs in question 2. Infrequently use intentionally (at times done unintentionally)	1. Never rechallenge potentially life-threatening drug reactions 2. Seldom rechallenge reaction with significant morbidity 3. Perform if no suitable alternative exits for potentially serious disease
Exclusion	1. Exclude nondrug causes of reaction pattern 2. Exclude systemic aspects of drug reaction	1. Some nondrug causes not easily diagnosed 2. Some drug reaction systemic components may be delayed
Additional FDA criteria		
Biologic plausibility	Mechanism of drug correlates with drug reaction mechanism	Most drug reactions do not have clear-cut mechanism
Class effect	Members of a drug class typically cross-react	Tetracyclines in particular differ in types of reactions
Dose relationship	Subtoxic doses often correlate with likelihood of reaction	Most reactions without clear dose correlation

Abbreviation: FDA, Food and Drug Administration.

- *Exclusion*: this prospective step includes excluding other etiologies for the same clinical presentation (ruling out viral hepatitis in patients with possible drug-induced liver injury) and testing for systemic aspects of a given clinical presentation (eg, testing for hematologic, liver, renal, and thyroid elements of DRESS syndrome)

Kramer Criteria

The Kramer criteria consist of the following: definite (all four criteria positive), probable (all criteria positive except rechallenge), possible (only challenge criteria positive plus either dechallenge or exclusion step), and unlikely (only challenge criteria positive).[17,18] In most clinical settings with drug reactions (aside from somewhat expected systemic adverse effects, such as cyclosporine-induced chronic kidney injury) clinicians work in the possible and unlikely realm of relatively low certainty.

The U.S. Food and Drug Administration (FDA) routinely uses other diagnostic components in addition to the previous algorithm to sort out cases reported to this agency.

- Biologic plausibility: correlating the drug mechanism with the drug reaction mechanism (statins inducing ichthyosis caused by epidermal cholesterol depletion).[19]
- Class effect: concept that members of the same drug class often produce similar drug reactions through cross-reaction (eg, various β-lactam antibiotics inducing urticarial reactions; various aromatic anticonvulsants, such as phenytoin, phenobarbital, and carbamazepine, inducing SJS/TEN and DRESS syndrome reactions).[6–9]
- Dose relationship: concept that a higher dose of a given drug is more likely to induce a drug reaction (eg, MTX-induced fatty liver/cirrhosis is more likely with higher cumulative doses).[20] In reality, most drug reactions do not have a strong dose correlation.

POTENTIAL PITFALLS OF THIS CLINICAL ALGORITHM

Limitations are next discussed for each step of the Kramer-FDA combined algorithm.

Challenge Step

The literature reputation of the suspected drug is unclear as with inflammatory bowel disease (IBD) and isotretinoin.[21] Delayed timing: most acute drug-induced liver injury occurs from 15 to 90 days; it is uncommon for the most serious acute drug reactions to occur after 3 months.[22,23]

Dechallenge Step

There is partial or no resolution of the drug reaction. A sine wave-like waxing and waning is characteristic of most autoimmune diseases. This makes clarifying which drugs that may induce or treat this category of disease difficult. There is prolonged half-life in serum or tissue as with etretinate storage in fat up to 2.9 years.[24]

Rechallenge Step

Rechallenge is not realistic or safe in most clinical settings for possible drug reactions (see **Table 3**). Rechallenge should be performed only if (1) the drug reaction is not even possibly life-threatening, (2) no suitable chemically unrelated drug alternatives are available, and (3) there is caution with even moderate-risk (non–life threatening) reactions with significant potential morbidity.

Exclusion Steps

Rule out other causes for the same clinical presentation (eg, viral vs drug-induced morbilliform reactions have no specific prompt reliable testing for most viral exanthems). Several of the systemic elements of cutaneous drug reactions with systemic features are delayed, such as hypothyroidism in patients with DRESS syndrome.

Biologic Plausibility

Specific mechanisms for most drug reaction patterns are not well-defined. Specific mechanisms for the drugs suspected in causing specific drug reactions are generally not well-defined.

Class Effect

Minocycline can induce DRESS syndrome, serum-sickness-like reaction, and drug-induced lupus, whereas other tetracycline family members including doxycycline do not induce any of these unique reactions.[25] Lamotrigine is not an aromatic anticonvulsant, but potentially coreacts inducing SJS/TEN and DRESS syndrome.[6–9] Gabapentin was developed as an anticonvulsant, yet has no significant risk of SJS/TEN or DRESS syndrome.

Dose Relationship

Most drug reactions in all three broad categories discussed are not dose-related and can occur at subtoxic and even subtherapeutic dose ranges.

THE BOTTOM-LINE: CAN THE DRUG/DRUGS IN QUESTION BE CONTINUED AND/OR RESTARTED

From a practical standpoint, all the prior information (principles and exceptions) boils down to a clinician's choice whether the drug/drugs in question can be discontinued, and can the drug/drugs in question be used (rechallenged) in the future subsequent to the drug reaction clinical resolution. The risk of drug continuation and/or rechallenge is the most important factor driving this drug reaction decision process.

Two clinical scenarios illustrate this process.[8,9] In drug-induced morbilliform reaction without features of DRESS syndrome and likely caused by a drug not characteristically inducing DRESS syndrome in a patient receiving the drug in question for chemotherapy, if no chemically unrelated suitable alternatives are available, it is reasonable to continue the drug in question under careful observation. If the previous clinical scenario involves instead a DRESS syndrome with a drug well-documented to induce DRESS syndrome, clinical wisdom is to promptly discontinue the drug in question because of the potentially life-threatening elements of the severe drug reaction and vigorously manage the clinical features of DRESS syndrome.

The critical feature of these scenarios is the magnitude of risk of the specific drug reaction suspected. In general, drug continuation or rechallenge is best avoided in higher risk drug reactions as follows: cutaneous drug reactions with systemic features (see **Table 1**); systemic reactions of potentially life-threatening features (see **Table 1**); and in both categories of drug reactions, a clinical decision generally must be made with far less than 100% certainty.

SOME ADDITIONAL PITFALLS BEYOND THE CLINICAL ALGORITHM

The following are some additional diagnostic pitfalls beyond the limitations of the clinical algorithm.

- Assumption that most drug reaction timing resembles that of type I hypersensitivity reactions, such as urticarial drug eruptions with initial sensitization in 7 to 14 days after the drug is started, and with rechallenge, the reaction occurs within minutes to hours or at latest a few days. The minority of drug reaction mechanisms, when known, are caused by type I hypersensitivity.
- Given the previously mentioned realities, eosinophils in tissue on hematoxylin and eosin are consistently involved in just type I hypersensitivity (and not types II through IV hypersensitivity) and have a central role in DRESS syndrome (largely of unknown mechanism). Tissue eosinophils are overrated in drug reaction diagnosis.
- Most drug reactions in the second and third categories in **Table 1** are believed caused by metabolic idiosyncratic mechanisms, which tend to peak between 3 and 8 weeks, and most occur within 3 months after drug initiation.[22,23]
- Patch testing for drug reaction diagnosis presumes the drug reaction is based on type IV hypersensitivity as with allergic contact dermatitis. Aside from diagnosing systemic contact dermatitis (type IV hypersensitivity) and perhaps morbilliform reactions there is little evidence that patch testing precisely helps diagnose most drug reactions discussed in this article.[26]

PITFALLS WHEN INTERPRETING THE LITERATURE INTERPRETATION

The topic of interpretation of the medical literature is vast and beyond the scope of this article. However, there are a few general principles and limitations of literature interpretation and regulatory agency response worth emphasizing.

- The pyramid detailing the hierarchy of evidence when interpreting scientific literature generally provides limited certainty in the diagnosis of cutaneous drug reactions.[27] In most scenarios either studies with higher levels of evidence are quite uncommon with drug reaction diagnosis, or most clinical reports are at the level of case reports and small case series.
- In these case reports and case series, a wide variation exists on the level of certainty based on information reported applied to the Kramer criteria (discussed previously).
- Many lists of drug causation in review articles or textbooks do not list specific references defining the reason for inclusion in the list provided.
- A warning and boxed warning (the latter is also known as black box warning) reported by the FDA are statements of potential risk and are not required to definitively establish causation before publication.
- It is a common event on various media to promptly see medical-legal law firms run advertisements for potential clients once warnings are communicated by the FDA; these warnings do not require establishment of a causal role for the drug (or product) in question.

- At times, there is a pendulum of the literature where alternately causation is tentatively established, followed by subsequent articles excluding to a reasonable degree this causal relationship. The long saga of the possible relationship between isotretinoin and IBD is an example.[21]
- There are times when larger epidemiologic studies show no causal role for a drug/adverse event (AE) combination, but individual cases have been reported for which the causation algorithm reaches the highest level by the Kramer criteria. This possibility is illustrated by a small subset of isotretinoin patients experiencing significant depression that promptly resolves when isotretinoin is discontinued (I have personally observed this).

PITFALLS OF PERSONAL EXPERIENCE

It is common for academicians and private practitioners in all fields of medicine to somewhat authoritatively mention the following two phrases. Some potential counterpoints follow each phrase.

"I have seen that before"
- Faulty causation algorithm possibly is used; very commonly there is a positive challenge step only with suboptimal timing with drug initiation of over 3 months previously.
- All of us are potentially susceptible to internal biases and personal areas of interest that may skew the true incidence of what we have "seen before."
- It is of great importance, however, to learn from previous clinical experience with drug reactions (even with low to moderate level of certainty of causation).
"I have not seen that before"
- From a statistical standpoint, a single clinician would need to see three times the incidence number for a specific drug AE to have statistical significance of personally not seeing the AE before.[28]
- For example, if the true incidence of severe ketoconazole hepatotoxicity is 1 in 10,000 a clinician would need to treat 30,000 patients with ketoconazole to have statistical significance to one's personal clinical experience.
- There are three potential modifiers to the previous scenario involving ketoconazole: (1) short ketoconazole courses for one or two doses fall short of the characteristic 15- to 90-day time frame for drug-induced hepatotoxicity and most important hypersensitivity reactions; (2) careful monitoring of transaminases may prevent more serious hepatotoxicity; and (3) careless (or no) monitoring might miss more moderate hepatotoxicity, which can be asymptomatic (this is more likely with azathioprine and dapsone use for which many clinicians just focus on hematologic monitoring).

SOME STATISTICAL PRINCIPLES OF VALUE IN EPIDEMIOLOGIC STUDY INTERPRETATION

There are two statistical measures that can assist the interpretation of epidemiologic studies.[29,30] Attributable risk (AR) is the incidence of a given outcome (drug AE in this case) minus the background or placebo incidence rate. AR is generally expressed in decimal form. Large clinical trials, case-control epidemiologic studies, registries, and systematic reviews or meta-analyses are capable of generating a meaningful AR. In each case, denominator data are essential to calculate this statistic.

Number needed to harm (NNH) is a more practical statistic to determine how many patients need to be treated with a specific drug to develop a specific AE. This statistic is calculated in whole numbers using similar studies to determine the AR. Statistically, the formula is $1/AR = NNH$. Some examples are listed next.

- NNH for azithromycin cardiovascular sudden death (AR = 0.00005) NNH = 19,142, thus a distinctly rare event.
- NNH for azithromycin cardiovascular sudden death is (AR = 0.00025) NNH = 4081 when studying the population with the highest decile of risk.[31–33]
- NNH for isotretinoin and IBD is (AR = 0.00034) NNH = 2977 initially[34] and subsequently (AR = 0.00019) NNH = 5130.[35] The latter study had an NNH that was statistically equal to the background rate of IBD, thus not reaching significance.
- Early studies suggested a risk of IBD,[36] whereas later studies did not show any significant risk.[37]

The NNH statistic is particularly useful when a hazard ratio is relatively high for a rare AE in the treatment of a common disease. It provides an understandable (to the patient) risk statistic when prescribing an important drug for the patient, such as isotretinoin for scarring acne.

SUMMARY

Clinical practice decisions are made many times daily using less than ideal data; it will always be that way in clinical practice. The information presented in this article helps clinicians attain the highest possible level of certainty before making these clinical decisions. Communication of this relative uncertainty to the patient, and more importantly what measures will be taken to minimize the risks discussed, is satisfactory for most patients.

REFERENCES

1. Gerson D, Sriganeshan V, Alexis JB. Cutaneous drug eruptions: a 5-year experience. J Am Acad Dermatol 2008;59(6):995–9.
2. Shiohara T. Fixed drug eruption: pathogenesis and diagnostic tests [Review]. Curr Opin Allergy Clin Immunol 2009;9(4):316–21.
3. Sehgal VN, Srivastava G. Fixed drug eruption (FDE): changing scenario of incriminating drugs [Review]. Int J Dermatol 2006;45(8):897–908.
4. Fortuna G, Salas-Alanis JC, Guidetti E, et al. A critical reappraisal of the current data on drug-induced linear immunoglobulin A bullous dermatosis: a real and separate nosological entity? [Review]. J Am Acad Dermatol 2012;66(6):988–94.
5. Onodera H, Mihm MC Jr, Yoshida A, et al. Drug-induced linear IgA bullous dermatosis [Review]. J Dermatol 2005;32(9):759–64.
6. Schwartz RA, McDonough PH, Lee BW. Toxic epidermal necrolysis: part I. Introduction, history, classification, clinical features, systemic manifestations, etiology, and immunopathogenesis [Review]. J Am Acad Dermatol 2013;69(2):173.e1–13 [quiz: 185–6].
7. Schwartz RA, McDonough PH, Lee BW. Toxic epidermal necrolysis: part II. Prognosis, sequelae, diagnosis, differential diagnosis, prevention, and treatment [Review]. J Am Acad Dermatol 2013; 69(2):187.e1–16 [quiz: 203–4].
8. Husain Z, Reddy BY, Schwartz RA. DRESS syndrome: part I. Clinical perspectives [Review]. J Am Acad Dermatol 2013;68(5):693.e1–14 [quiz: 706–8].
9. Husain Z, Reddy BY, Schwartz RA. DRESS syndrome: part II. Management and therapeutics [Review]. J Am Acad Dermatol 2013;68(5):709.e1–9 [quiz: 718–20].
10. Bailey K, McKee D, Wismer J, et al. Acute generalized exanthematous pustulosis induced by hydroxychloroquine: first case report in Canada and review of the literature [Review]. J Cutan Med Surg 2013; 17(6):414–8.
11. Fernando SL. Acute generalized exanthematous pustulosis [Review]. Australas J Dermatol 2012; 53(2):87–92.
12. Callen JP, Kulp-Shorten CL. Methotrexate. In: Wolverton SE, editor. Comprehensive dermatologic drug therapy. 3rd edition. Philadelphia: WB Saunders; 2012. p. 169–81.
13. Bhutani T, Lee CS, Koo JYM. Cyclosporine. In: Wolverton SE, editor. Comprehensive dermatologic drug therapy. 3rd edition. Philadelphia: WB Saunders; 2012. p. 199–211.
14. Perrillo RP, Martin P, Lok AS. Preventing hepatitis B reactivation due to immunosuppressive drug treatments. JAMA 2015;313(16):1617–8.
15. Di Bisceglie AM, Lok AS, Martin P, et al. Recent US Food and Drug Administration warnings on hepatitis B reactivation with immune-suppressing and anti-cancer drugs: just the tip of the iceberg? [Review]. Hepatology 2015;61(2):703–11.
16. Wolverton SE, Remlinger K. Suggested guidelines for patient monitoring: hepatic and hematologic toxicity attributable to systemic dermatologic drugs [Review]. Dermatol Clin 2007;25(2):195–205, vi–vii.
17. Kramer MS, Leventhal JM, Hutchinson TA, et al. An algorithm for the operational assessment of adverse drug reactions. I. Background, description, and instructions for use. JAMA 1979;242(7):623–32.
18. Vaisrub S. Groping for causation [Editorial]. JAMA 1979;241(8):830.
19. Goldberg I, Isman G, Shirazi I, et al. Interferon-gamma (INF-gamma) release test can detect cutaneous adverse effects to statins. Int J Dermatol 2009;48(12):1370–5.
20. Menter A, Korman NJ, Elmets CA, et al. Guidelines of care for the management of psoriasis and psoriatic arthritis: section 4. Guidelines of care for the management and treatment of psoriasis with traditional systemic agents. J Am Acad Dermatol 2009; 61(3):451–85.
21. Wolverton SE, Harper JC. Important controversies associated with isotretinoin therapy for acne [Review]. Am J Clin Dermatol 2013;14(2):71–6.
22. Zimmerman HJ, Ishak KG. General aspects of drug-induced liver disease. Gastroenterol Clin North Am 1995;24:739–57.
23. Wolverton SE. Major adverse effects from systemic drugs: defining the risks. Curr Probl Dermatol 1995;7:1–40.
24. Wiegand UW, Chou RC. Pharmacokinetics of acitretin and etretinate. J Am Acad Dermatol 1998;39: S25–33.
25. Lebrun-Vignes B, Kreft-Jais C, Castot A, et al, French Network of Regional Centers of Pharmacovigilance. Comparative analysis of adverse drug reactions to tetracyclines: results of a French national survey and review of the literature [Review]. Br J Dermatol 2012;166(6):1333–41.
26. Friedmann PS, Ardern-Jones M. Patch testing in drug allergy [Review]. Curr Opin Allergy 2010;10(4):291–6.
27. Rosner AL. Evidence-based medicine: revisiting the pyramid of priorities [Review]. J Bodyw Mov Ther 2012;16(1):42–9.
28. Gelfand JM, Langan SM. Pharmacovigilance: verifying that drugs remain safe. In: Wolverton SE, editor. Comprehensive dermatologic drug therapy. 3rd edition. Philadelphia: WB Saunders; 2012. p. 46–53.

29. Citrome L. Relative vs. absolute measures of benefit and risk: what's the difference? Acta Psychiatr Scand 2010;121(2):94–102.

30. Altman DG. Confidence intervals for the number needed to treat. BMJ 1998;317:1309–12.

31. Ray WA, Murray KT, Hall K, et al. Azithromycin and the risk of cardiovascular death. N Engl J Med 2012;366:1881–90.

32. Svanstrom H, Pasternak B, Hviid A. Use of azithromycin and death from cardiovascular causes. N Engl J Med 2013;368:1704–12.

33. Mosholder AD, Mathew J, Alexander JJ, et al. Cardiovascular risks with azithromycin and other antibacterial drugs. N Engl J Med 2013;368:1665–8.

34. Popescu CM, Popescu R. Isotretinoin therapy and inflammatory bowel disease. Arch Dermatol 2011; 147(6):724–9.

35. Popescu CM, Bigby M. The weight of evidence on the association of isotretinoin use and the development of inflammatory bowel disease. JAMA Dermatol 2013;149(2):221–2.

36. Reddy D, Siegel CA, Sands BE, et al. Possible association between isotretinoin and inflammatory bowel disease. Am J Gastroenterol 2006;101:1569–73.

37. Alhusayen RO, Juurlink DN, Mamdani MM, et al. Isotretinoin use and the risk of inflammatory bowel disease: a population-based study. J Invest Dermatol 2012;133(4):907–12.

Practice and Educational Gaps in Radiation Therapy in Dermatology

Armand B. Cognetta Jr, MD[a], Christopher M. Wolfe, DO[a],*,
David J. Goldberg, MD, JD[b,c], Hyokyoung Grace Hong, PhD[d]

KEYWORDS

- Superficial radiation treatment • Superficial radiotherapy • Dermatologic radiotherapy
- Nonmelanoma skin cancer • Basal cell carcinoma • Squamous cell carcinoma
- Treatment selection criteria • Appropriate use criteria

KEY POINTS

- Superficial radiation therapy has more than 106 years of research and development by dermatologists.
- Compared with hospital-based radiation therapy delivered by radiation oncologists, superficial radiation delivered in the outpatient dermatologic setting is the least expensive form of radiation treatment.
- Superficial radiation therapy is currently an underused modality in the treatment of nonmelanoma skin cancer.
- With the aging, feeble population it is vital to keep this cost-efficient modality within the hands of dermatologists.

Superficial radiation therapy (SRT) has been the standard of care for office-based radiation treatment of nonmelanoma skin cancers (NMSC) for more than 100 years. This began with Leopold Freund (acknowledged as the father of radiation therapy [RT]), with a continuous lineage from him to Pusey, MacKee, Cippolaro, Goldsmith, Gladstein, Panizzon, and Kopf. SRT was an integral part of dermatology practices for the better part of the 20th century until the mid 1980s, when the popularity of Mohs surgery and the cessation of manufacturing of new and modern SRT platforms led to a decrease in the popularity of SRT. An American Academy of Dermatology (AAD) task force in 1974 concluded that 55% of dermatology offices used SRT and 44% of dermatologists used SRT regularly.

The physics of SRT are less complex than any laser/light platform in use by dermatologists today. X-rays are part of the electromagnetic spectrum beginning just beyond the ultraviolet spectrum. Dermatologists have embraced and pioneered use of the entire electromagnetic spectrum. From conception, design, and fine tuning, to use, SRT remains within the purview of dermatologic therapy. Dermatologists consider themselves

Funding Sources: None.
Conflicts of Interest: None.
Disclosures: A.B. Cognetta served as an unpaid advisor for Topex (now Sensus Healthcare) and was given a stock option for his advisory role.
[a] Division of Dermatology, Florida State University College of Medicine, Tallahassee, FL, USA; [b] Skin Laser & Surgery Specialists of NY and NJ, USA; [c] Department of Dermatology, Mt. Sinai School of Medicine, New York, NY, USA; [d] Department of Statistics and Probability, Michigan State University, East Lansing, MI, USA
* Corresponding author. 604 Tree Duck Court, Greensburg, PA 15601.
E-mail address: wolfe1pa@gmail.com

Dermatol Clin 34 (2016) 319–333
http://dx.doi.org/10.1016/j.det.2016.02.011
0733-8635/16/$ – see front matter © 2016 Elsevier Inc. All rights reserved.

derm.theclinics.com

cutaneous oncologists, using imaging, targeted therapy, immunotherapy, surgery, and primary as well as adjunctive radiotherapy to treat skin cancer. With the aging, feeble population it is vital to keep this cost-efficient modality within the hands of dermatologists.

Dermatology has played a pivotal role in the conception and development of many other subspecialties such as rheumatology, venereology, cosmetic surgery, and radiation oncology. Long before the American Club of Therapeutic Radiologists was formed in 1962, (the precursor to the American Society for Therapeutic Radiology and Oncology [ASTRO]),[1] dermatologists were pioneering the use of RT and brachytherapy. A de facto relinquishment of SRT to radiation oncologists would be comparable with (1) relinquishment of laser therapy to plastic surgeons because it falls within the realm of cosmetic treatment, (2) Mohs surgery to general and plastic surgeons simply because it is surgery, or (3) dermatopathology to general pathologists.

BEST PRACTICES IN DERMATOLOGIC RADIOTHERAPY

Best practice includes consensus development based on best evidence formulated by dermatologists with the most experience using a particular radiation modality. This practice includes the creation of a treatment algorithm for NMSC and incorporation of SRT into the treatment algorithm for the population over the age of 65. At present, guidelines exist based on past research, though no appropriate use criteria (AUC) have been developed. The most critical aspect of SRT use is appropriate patient and tumor selection.

The following are proposed SRT AUC for basal cell carcinoma (BCC)/squamous cell carcinoma (SCC) treatment that are accepted by experienced dermatology radiotherapists in the past and present:

1. Location: central face, including the eyelids, nasal tip, nasal ala, ears, lips.[2–34]
2. Age ≥60 years: to minimize the synergistic effects of ultraviolet radiation and late sequelae.[35–40]
3. Tumor size: tumors up to 5 cm in diameter may be adequately treated with SRT.[10,41–45]
4. Tumor type/depth of invasion: superficial and nodular BCCs, SCC in situ, and SCC that are nonaggressive are amenable to SRT.[6,42,43,46]
5. Frailty and medical status: inability to tolerate surgery owing to poor health, multiple comorbidities, or those on anticoagulant therapy may have a higher risk of adverse surgical

events. Eastern Cooperative Oncology Group performance status[47] may be used to document selection of radiotherapy over surgery.
6. Patient preference to avoid surgery may be a consideration and in cases where surgery will lead to skin graft or complex flap closure.

Absolute (1–4) and relative (5,6) contraindications for SRT include the following:

1. Aggressive tumor histology: BCCs (sclerosing, morpheaform, infiltrative), SCC (perineural invasion, arising in previous sites of RT, burn scars, chronic ulcers, spindle cell carcinoma, poorly/undifferentiated, or those secondary to osteomyelitis).[6,42,43,46,48–51]
2. Deep tumor invasion: tumors that invade bone, cartilage, or arise within the mucosal surfaces (intranasal/intraoral).[52,53]
3. Previously irradiated site: increases incidence of late-term sequelae (ulcer, radionecrosis of cartilage and bone) results in unsatisfactory cosmesis, recurrence, and second primary tumors.[48,49,54,55]
4. Genetic anomalies: nevoid BCC syndrome, xeroderma pigmentosum, Garner's syndrome, Li-Fraumeni syndrome, and others with increased radiosensitivity or where radiation may induce new malignancies.[56–63]
5. Organ transplant recipients: the mainstay of treatment is surgical excision or Mohs surgery.
6. Location on the trunk or extremities: early pioneers of SRT recommended against the use of radiotherapy on the trunk and extremities owing to late sequelae changes (telengiectasias and pigmentary changes), lower oxygen saturation leading to potential decreased efficacy and wound healing issues, and the general ease and expediency of surgical removal.[44,64–69]

ESTIMATE OF CURRENT PRACTICE

The 1974 AAD Task Force on Ionizing Radiation conducted a comprehensive survey sending a detailed questionnaire to 4560 dermatologists in the United States and Canada. Of the 2444 replies, 44% of respondents (1075) reported using radiotherapy weekly.[70] Superficial x-ray or Grenz-ray equipment was reported to be available in 55.5% of dermatologic offices. A larger pool of dermatologists in the past had considerable experience with the use of in-office radiotherapy and helped to shape, by their use and research, the guidelines in use today. Recently, there has been a noticeable resurgence in the interest and use of SRT by dermatologists with the reintroduction of more modern, user-friendly, and safer equipment.

Research is currently being undertaken to ascertain current SRT utilization rates.

PRACTICE GAPS IN THE USE OF SUPERFICIAL RADIATION THERAPY IN CLINICAL DERMATOLOGY PRACTICE
Knowledge Gap Within Dermatology Professional Organizations

In a 2013 position statement, the AAD grouped newer technologies such as high-dose electronic brachytherapy (EBT), together with SRT as a "new" therapy with the need for "research on long-term outcomes." The AAD has since clarified these modalities in an addendum position statement. Nonetheless, the AAD continues to mistakenly refer to SRT as a "new" technology that "differs substantially from traditional external beam radiation therapy" and one in need of "research on long term outcomes." This is despite the fact that SRT was the standard radiation modality in use by dermatologists long before electron beam therapy was conceived or used. Goldschmidt in his 1978 book "Physical Modalities in Dermatologic Therapy" reports that superficial x-ray machines were the most commonly used dermatologic radiotherapy units in the United States and Canada in 1975.[70] Similarly, long-term SRT outcomes have been reported in the past and continue to be reported by dermatologists.[2–27,30,44–46,50,64,65,68,71–110]

Perceived Research Gaps

SRT has more than a century's worth of research and development. Dermatologists were the first radiation oncologists applying SRT to treat skin disease as early as 1897, shortly after the discovery of x-rays by Wilhelm C. Roentgen in 1895, and decades before the specialties of radiology and radiation oncology emerged and then diverged. Pioneers in radiotherapy, dermatologists authored, and more recently coauthored with radiation oncologists, textbooks that have been in continuous publication since 1921 on the use of SRT and radium in skin disease.[67,82,109–113] The first reported results using radiotherapy came from dermatologists in what was the precursor to the annual AAD meeting, "Rationale of and the Indications for Therapeutic Use of Rontgen Rays" (27th Annual Meeting of the American Dermatological Association, Washington, May 13th and 14th, 1903).

Dermatologists were the first to look at fractionation and its effects on early and late sequelae.[77,78] Dermatologists formulated fractionation schemes[65,88,112,114,115] and time dose fractionation formulas[116–121] enabling treatment plan optimization. They were the first to incorporate the $D_{1/2}$ concept to ensure adequate depth radiation dose to the tumor base.[50,122–124] The body of knowledge and experience that we have inherited from our predecessors in dermatologic radiotherapy is immense and still valid today.

The Randomized, Clinical Trials Conundrum Gap

The AAD in their recent Position Statement on SRT and Electronic Brachytherapy for BCC and SCC disallowed all studies that were not randomized, clinical trials (RCTs). Of note, authors Levy and Stasko in Alams' book "Evidenced-Based Procedural Dermatology"[125] uncovered only 2 RCTs involving Mohs micrographic surgery, both comparing Mohs micrographic surgery with surgical excision.[126,127] They state that the bulk of literature regarding Mohs micrographic surgery consists of case studies, systematic reviews, and meta-analyses. They note that most of the literature on Mohs micrographic surgery is retrospective, nonrandomized, and suffers from selection bias. This is the same argument used by most critics of SRT, yet Mohs micrographic surgery is still accepted as the treatment of choice for NMSC in many situations.

The authors report that "the level of risk for a type of skin cancer often drives the decision of which treatment is used." It is on this basis, as well as patient factors, that SRT is offered to select patients/tumors. Similar to Mohs micrographic surgery, the vast majority of research that has formed the foundation of dermatologic radiotherapy has come from retrospective analysis of patients chosen for SRT. From these studies we have gained an in-depth understanding of optimal dosimetry based on tumor characteristics and patient factors.[2–9,11,12,14–34,45,64,68,73,83,84,91–104,106,112,128–132]

Randomized trials for the treatment of skin cancer are near impossible to undertake. To assign patients randomly to various modalities today would increase significantly the risk of recurrence, morbidity, and even mortality. For example, megavoltage RT is often used as a primary treatment or adjunct to surgery for tumors invading bone and orbital structures; however, one would never randomize a cohort of patients with carcinoma invading bone to Mohs surgery versus treatment with RT alone.

An additional argument against SRT is that studies involving RT should confirm the long-term clearance of residual tumor based on histologic analysis of the irradiated tissue several years later. This unnecessary step, in light of clinical follow-up, further subjects the patient to increased morbidity by excision or multiple random biopsies. We could uncover no studies that follow NMSC surgery patients for 5 years then re-excise the scar created from the initial surgery to histologically confirm the absence of residual tumor. The expectation that this should be done with RT is equally implausible.

National Comprehensive Cancer Network Guidelines Gap

The National Comprehensive Cancer Network (NCCN) established guidelines for the treatment of NMSC to include RT; however, only electron beam RT and orthovoltage RT, performed by radiation oncologists, are included in the consensus guidelines.[48,49] These guidelines fail to mention SRT as a modality to treat NMSC. Of the 28 panel members that developed the NMSC NCCN guidelines, 16 are dermatologists (10 Mohs surgeons), 5 are medical oncologists, 5 are surgical oncologists, 1 is a pathology trained dermatopathologist, and 1 is a radiation oncologist.

Use Gap

In 1981, Goldschmidt[83] noted that RT had been used routinely in the treatment of 10% to 20% of skin cancers in leading dermatologic institutions where all other forms of therapy were also available. Goldschmidt noted that 400,000 new cases of skin cancer were occurring each year in the United States (1981); if dermatologists were to cease using ionizing radiation, 40,000 to 80,000 patients would have to be treated with other modalities that may not have been the treatment of choice, such as surgery or more expensive RT modalities (**Table 1**).[83]

The senior author estimates that 500 SRT units are in use across the United States. With about 10,000 actively practicing dermatologists, 1 out of 20 dermatologists (5%) are offering this modality as a treatment option. Based on our own experience, 5% of patients diagnosed with, or referred for, NMSC treatment are eligible for and choose treatment with SRT. Extrapolated this represents a 0.25% overall use of SRT by dermatologists, whereas 5% is likely an optimal use rate.

We surveyed a random sample of dermatologists practicing in the United States regarding their use of SRT for the treatment of skin cancer. Of 67 respondents, 60 (90%) stated they did not use radiotherapy in their office on a weekly basis and 58 of the 67 (87%) did not have radiation equipment available. Only 15 of the 67 (22%) reported an SRT use rate of 1% to 5% for BCC treatment and 50 of the 67 (75%) reported no use at all for BCC. Only 13 (19%) reported an SRT utilization

Table 1
Radiotherapy cost comparison

Treatment Method	Total Cost to Treat Including Recurrences
Mohs micrographic surgery: nose/eyelid with FTSG repair	1767.50 $US
Mohs micrographic surgery: nose/eyelid with flap repair	1670.60 $US
Dermatologic office-based radiation (5 fractions) used in our practice	687.38 $US
Dermatologic office-based superficial radiation (12 fractions)	1019.20 $US
High-dose rate electronic brachytherapy (8 fractions)	8046.86 $US
Hospital-based orthovoltage radiation (20 fractions)	3889.80 $US
Hospital-based megavoltage radiation/electron beam (20 fractions)	7281.79 $US

Abbreviation: FTSG, full-thickness skin graft.

rate of 1% to 5% for SCC treatment and 53 (79%) reported no use for SCC. These responses are in line with our hypothesis that SRT is underused in the treatment of NMSC. Research is currently being undertaken to ascertain rates of use from Medicare data.

Radiation Therapy Terminology Knowledge Gap

The AAD Position Statement on SRT and EBT for BCC and SCC exemplifies the confusion that exists between various x-ray platforms. The original intent of EBT manufacturers was to provide intracavitary placement of miniaturized cathodes deep in tumor beds for neoplasms such as breast cancer where the delivery of high-dose photons is done only once before surgical closure of the wound. EBT systems use no radioactive gamma-emitting isotopes; they use a conventional but miniaturized x-ray tube that emits a multispectral beam of photon radiation. With a source to surface distance that ranges between 2.5 and 6 cm, EBT may be characterized more appropriately as contact therapy radiation or ultrashort distance radiotherapy. Early predecessors of these x-ray machines (Chaoul and Philips units), with a source to surface distance of 1.5 to 3.0 cm, were in existence in the late 1940s and are still in use today[81,133] (**Figs. 1** and **2**).

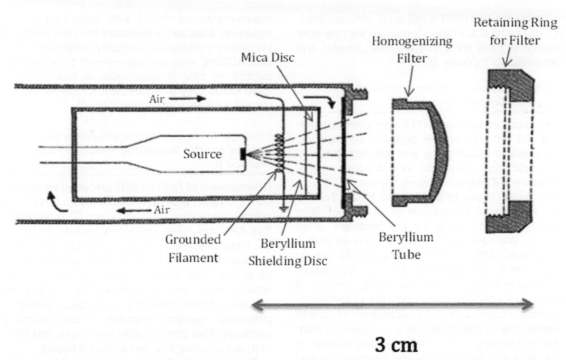

Fig. 1. Philips RT 50: "Contact" therapy (Era 1950).

3 cm

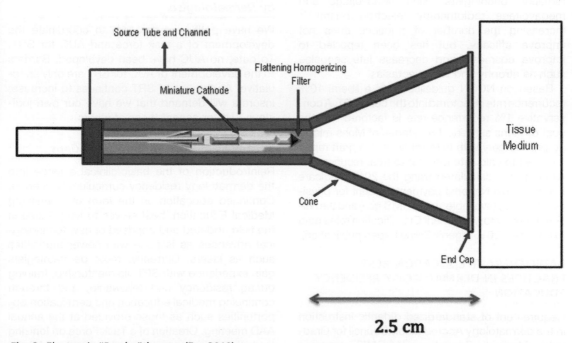

Fig. 2. Electronic "Brachy"therapy (Era 2010).

2.5 cm

Today, the term SRT is still used, although modern units emit soft x-rays. Compared with the older superficial x-ray units, they are safer, simpler, and more reliable[65] (**Table 2**).

Perceived Expense of Dermatology Office-based Radiotherapy Gap

Prior cost comparisons of RT in dermatologic literature did not differentiate between dermatologic office-based radiotherapy and radiation delivered by a radiation oncologist in a hospital setting. Rogers and Coldiron[134] report the cost of RT for a BCC on the cheek to be $2591 to $3460. **Table 3** presents a cost comparison of all RT modalities currently in use today for the treatment of an NMSC. We have calculated the costs to treat a T1-2N0M0 NMSC on the nose or eyelid, 2 locations SRT finds its greatest utility. The cost of Mohs micrographic surgery is calculated using 2 stages of Mohs micrographic surgery and a flap or graft repair (primary closure is often not possible on the nose or eyelid). The number of stages is derived from Alam and colleagues,[135] who reported the number of stages by anatomic location and geographic region for Mohs surgeons across the United States. The average number of stages was 1.96 for the periorbital region and 2.01 for the nose.[135] The multiple surgery reduction rule was applied.

Cost for RT is based on modality, location (hospital versus outpatient), and fractionation schedule. Reported fractionation includes 5 to 12 for SRT,[13,14] 8 for high-dose EBT,[136] and 20 by radiation oncologists using orthovoltage and megavoltage radiotherapy (electron beam).[137] Increasing the number of fractions does not improve efficacy, but has been reported to improve cosmesis and decrease late sequelae such as atrophy and telengiectasias.

Based on NCCN guidelines,[42,43] a liberal 10% recurrence rate is factored into the cost of RT. A conservative 1% recurrence rate is factored into the cost of Mohs surgery. Two stages of Mohs micrographic surgery with full-thickness skin graft repair are used to calculate the cost to treat recurrences. All costs are calculated using the 2015 Medicare Fee schedule National payment amount for physician services (available: www.CMS.gov) and the National Ambulatory Payment Classification rates paid to hospitals (2015 Ingenix Billing Expert publication).

RADIOTHERAPY EDUCATION BEST PRACTICES IN DERMATOLOGY RESIDENCY EDUCATION

Requirement of standardized didactic instruction in the dermatology Accreditation Council for Graduate Medical Education (ACGME) program requirements combined with opportunities for hands-on experience represent the best practice in residency education. Currently, there is no specific ACGME program requirement for either didactics or clinical experience in radiotherapy; there exists only a requirement for dermatology-related subspecialty experiences.[138]

Strategy to Correct the Appropriate Use Criteria for the Superficial Radiation Therapy Practice Gap

Development of AUC for SRT preceded by formation of a Task Force on Radiation made up of AAD members who use SRT and other RT modalities. The AAD has been petitioned repeatedly to do so. Optimally, members from the United States and around the world who routinely use SRT would be on this panel, along with experienced representatives from general dermatology, cutaneous oncology, Mohs micrographic surgery, dermatopathology, geriatric dermatology, and radiation oncology. This configuration will ensure that SRT AUC are conservative and evidence based.

The core of the AUC approach should continue to be the Appropriateness Method developed jointly by the Rand Corporation and UCLA in the 1980s to measure overuse and underuse of medical and surgical interventions by determining relative risks and harms.[139]

Barriers to the Development of Appropriate Use Criteria for Superficial Radiation Therapy by Dermatologists

We have petitioned the AAD to coordinate the development of a task force and AUC for SRT. To date, no AUC have been developed. Barriers to the development of AUC for SRT are only speculative. As the use of SRT continues to increase, insurers will demand that we have our own judicious AUC or accept those of others.

Strategies to Correct Knowledge Gaps

Reintroduction of the basic/clinical science into the dermatology residency curriculum is needed. Continued education, in the form of Continuing Medical Education, best serves to keep those in the field updated and apprised of new technological advances as is done with newer modalities such as lasers. Currently, most dermatologists gain experience with SRT via mentorship, training during residency and fellowship, and through continuing medical education and certification opportunities such as those provided at the annual AAD meeting. Creation of a Task Force on Ionizing Radiation, which once existed within the AAD, by

Table 2
Radiation therapy terminology: Classification of radiotherapy methods based on energy/voltage/generator

Type	Sources and Synonyms	Type of Generator	kV	SSD (cm)	$D_{1/2}$ mm Tissue	Surface Dose (%)[a]
Megavoltage electron therapy	Electron beam radiation	LINAC	>1000 (6000–9000)	80	90% isodose method used for electrons[b]	78–86
Megavoltage photon therapy (not routinely used to treat NMSC)	Megavoltage X-ray	LINAC, Betatron	>1000	80	150–200	6–30
Supervoltage therapy	γ-ray	Isotope teletherapy Machines (60Cobalt)	400–800	50–80	80–110	40–90
Orthovoltage therapy	Deep x-ray	X-ray machine cathode	200–400	50–80	50–80	100
Intermediate therapy	Half-deep therapy	X-ray machine cathode	110–130	30	30	100
Contact therapy	Ultrashort distance (Chaoul)	X-ray machine cathode	50–60	1.5–3.0	4–30	100
Electronic brachytherapy[c]	Misnomer when used to treat skin cancer	Miniaturized cathode	50	2.5–6.0	3–7 (varies with probe position)	100
Superficial x-ray therapy[d]	Pyrex (glass) Window (older units),	X-ray machine cathode	60–100	15–30	7–20	100
Soft x-ray therapy[d]	Beryllium Window (modern units)	X-ray machine cathode	20–100	10–30	1–20	100
Grenz therapy	Ultrasoft therapy, supersoft therapy	X-ray machine cathode	5–20	10–15	0.2–0.8	100

Abbreviations: LINAC, linear accelerator; NMSC, nonmelanoma skin cancers; SSD, source to surface distance.
[a] Surface dose is the percent of radiation dose delivered to the skin surface.
[b] The 90% Isodose method is used by radiation or cologists for electron beam radiotherapy.
[c] Depth dose varies with position of the x-ray probe that is used.
[d] Superficial/soft x-ray therapy is the type most often used in dermatology office-based radiotherapy for squamous cell carcinoma, squamous cell carcinoma in situ, and basal cell carcinoma.

Adapted from Goldschmidt H. Treatment planning: selection of physical factors and radiation techniques. In: Goldschmidt H, Panizzon RG, editors. Modern dermatologic radiation therapy. New York: Springer-Verlag; 1991; p. 49–62; and Wolfe CM, Armand B. Cognetta J. Current use of dermatologic radiotherapy in the United States. In: Armand B, Cognetta J, Mendenhall WM, editors. Radiation therapy for skin cancer. New York: Springer; 2013:135; with permission.

Table 3
Residents desire for emphasis on radiation therapy in residency training programs in the future

Need for	More, n (%)	Same, n (%)	Less, n (%)	None, n (%)
Practical instruction	59 (75.64)	9 (11.54)	2 (2.56)	8 (10.26)
Theoretic instruction—indications	60 (76.92)	9 (11.54)	2 (2.56)	7 (8.97)
Theoretic instruction—techniques	56 (71.79)	11 (14.10)	3 (3.85)	8 (10.26)
Theoretic instruction—radiation physics	52 (66.67)	12 (15.38)	2 (2.56)	12 (15.38)

dermatologists that use SRT would prevent misinformation and steward appropriate use guidelines.

Strategies to Correct Perceived Research Gaps and the Randomized, Controlled Trial Conundrum

Inclusion of level II and III evidence with SRT for consensus and guideline development, as these studies provide important information about patient and tumor characteristics, recurrence rates, cosmetic outcomes, and other important data. It should be possible to design RCTs comparing various RT modalities for patients in whom RT is the appropriate choice based on patient and tumor factors—with randomization of these patients into cohorts receiving one of the various RT modalities such as SRT, orthovoltage, electron beam RT, or EBT. This type of randomization has been done previously in the 2 RCTs concerning Mohs micrographic surgery, both comparing Mohs surgery with simple excision.[126,127]

Strategies to Correct the National Comprehensive Cancer Network Guidelines Gap

To prevent perpetuating underlying bias introduced by members of original guideline panels, it has been suggested that periodic review by experts not involved with development of the initial guidelines be conducted.[140] Inclusion of at least 5 dermatologists who use both Mohs surgery and SRT as treatment options may help to prevent the exclusion of SRT by dermatologists from future NCCN guidelines. Development of future NCCN guidelines should include retrospective analyses of SRT. References for the recent NCCN guidelines for the treatment of BCC and SCC are derived mainly from retrospective studies, reviews of literature, and book chapters.[105,141–156] Two studies cited for defining high-risk features by location and size are retrospective analyses.[105,141] Of the 146 citations in the NCCN guidelines for both BCC and SCC, only 16 are randomized trials.[48,49] This analysis is not intended to discredit guideline recommendations, but is intended to illustrate that the majority of research for guideline development for treatment of BCC and SCC comes from retrospective analyses or meta-analyses.

Strategies to Correct the Use Gap

Calling on more than 70 specialty society partners including the AAD and ASTRO, the American Board of Internal Medicine Foundation launched "Choosing Wisely," a campaign to prevent unnecessary medical tests, treatments, and procedures through the promotion of conversations between clinicians and patients. The campaign is based on 4 tenets to help patients choose care that is (1) supported by evidence, (2) not duplicative of other tests or procedures already received, (3) free from harm, and (4) truly necessary. The key to "choosing wisely" with RT is to select therapy based on patient age, infirmity, comorbidities, tumor type and /depth, and patient choice. In line with choosing wisely, prospect theory is a concept applied to health values, which considers a patient's baseline functionality when determining the risk-to-benefit ratio for an intervention, acknowledges uncertainty, reflects patient's values, and allows for treatment that may not necessarily achieve the highest cure rate, but rather an acceptable one.

Conscious or unconscious, biases affect our medical decision making. Eaglstein[157] notes that several interlocking biases affect medical and surgical decision making, resulting in the underuse of effective therapies. Although SRT is often compared with and felt to be comparable with Mohs surgery and other surgical modalities, many if not most dermatologists fail to consider this form of treatment.

RADIOTHERAPY EDUCATION BEST PRACTICES IN DERMATOLOGY RESIDENCY EDUCATION

Requirement of standardized didactic instruction in dermatology residency ACGME program requirements, combined with opportunities for hands-on experience, represents the best practice in residency education. Currently, there is no specific ACGME program requirement for either didactics or clinical experience in radiotherapy.[138]

ESTIMATE OF CURRENT DERMATOLOGIC RADIOTHERAPY EDUCATION AND EDUCATIONAL GAPS

A survey of dermatologic training centers in the United States and Canada in 1986 by Kingery noted that only 12% used x-ray therapy and 81% included instruction in RT.[158] The most recent survey conducted by Schalock and colleagues[159] in 2005 sent surveys to 111 dermatology programs; 87 programs responded (78%) and only 10% of programs "have and use" x-ray or Grenz-ray equipment. However, 80% of dermatology programs included the theory and practice of RT in their curriculum.[159]

We surveyed residents of dermatology programs about their use of and instruction in RT. Out of 80 respondents, 79 (99%) reported that SRT equipment was not available for dermatology residents to treat skin cancer or that they did not know if it was available. Sixty-five percent (52/80) reported no didactic or practical exposure to SRT. Seventy-six percent (61/80) reported they did not feel prepared to discuss superficial/soft radiotherapy with patients as an option to treat their skin cancer. Fifty-nine percent (47/80) reported they would like to learn more about SRT as an alternative in the elderly and infirm. The majority of residents also reported a need for more instruction in RT (**Table 3**). These responses reveal both an education gap and a desire to learn more about SRT as a treatment option.

STRATEGIES TO CORRECT EDUCATIONAL GAPS IN DERMATOLOGY RESIDENCY EDUCATION

Review and standardization of the current radiotherapy curriculum in dermatology residencies by dermatologists experienced in the utilization of radiotherapy in conjunction with radiation physicists and other specialists in the field. This education could be in the form of basic science lectures incorporating dermatologist's use of the entire electromagnetic spectrum from infrared to gamma rays for the diagnosis and treatment of cutaneous disorders" (**Figs. 3** and **4**).

The curriculum should provide an understanding of the indications/limitations various forms of radiotherapy; SRT, EBT, and orthovoltage/megavoltage radiation delivered by radiation oncologists, when RT is chosen as the appropriate modality.

SUMMARY

SRT has more than 106 years' worth of research and development by dermatologists. One of the first reports on the use of radiotherapy came from dermatologists in 1903. Best practice consensus development and AUC based on best evidence established by dermatologists with the most experience using a particular radiation modality are warranted in light of "new" costly modalities that have begun to emerge. At present, general guidelines exist on appropriate use based

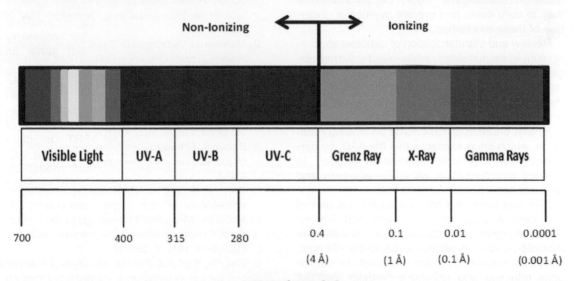

Fig. 3. The ionizing and nonionizing portions of the electromagnetic spectrum.

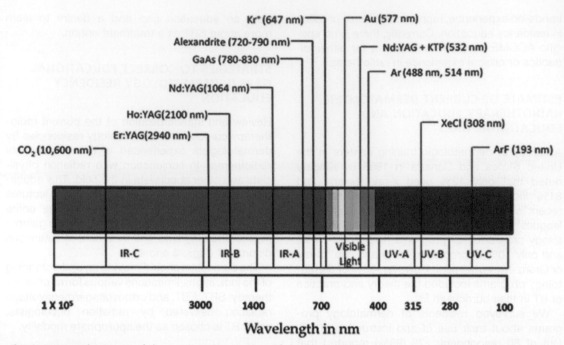

Fig. 4. Dermatologic use of the nonionizing portion of the electromagnetic spectrum. (*Adapted from* Steiner R. Basic laser physics. In: Raulin C and Karsai S, editors. Laser and IPL Technology in dermatology and aesthetic medicine. Berlin: Springer, 2010. p. 15; with permission.)

on prior research though no formal AUC have been developed.

AUC that cover patient selection, lesion selection, beam selection, and fractionation guidelines, and are formulated by multiple specialties including radiation oncologists, dermatologists, medical physicists, geriatricians, and Mohs surgeons, which applies to both dermatologists and radiation oncologists, would be an innovative way to curb costs and prevent overuse or underuse of these modalities.

Review and standardization of radiotherapy curriculum in dermatology residencies by dermatologists with experience in RT will alleviate misunderstanding and misinformation within the dermatology community and provide education and clinical experience for residents in RT.

Finally, creation of Task Force on Ionizing Radiation, which once existed within the AAD, by dermatologists that use radiation is needed to prevent misinformation within the academy and steward appropriate use guidelines.

SRT has been and remains an integral part of our dermatologic armamentarium and history. Although higher cure rates may possible with other modalities, there is always a risk-to-benefit analysis. This should never argue against dermatologists retaining and refining a modality that our predecessors developed nor should we limit its use by our successors. Most important, as the

least expensive form of RT, our elderly and infirm patients should continue to benefit from RT in outpatient dermatologic settings especially in light of the financial constraints on the healthcare system.

REFERENCES

1. Society History. Available at: www.astro.org/about-astro/society-history/index.aspx. Accessed May 5, 2015.
2. Mazeron JJ, Chassagne D, Crook J, et al. Radiation therapy of carcinomas of the skin of nose and nasal vestibule: a report of 1676 cases by the Groupe Europeen de Curietherapie. Radiother Oncol 1988;13(3):165–73.
3. Avila J, Bosch A, Aristizabal S, et al. Carcinoma of the pinna. Cancer 1977;40(6):2891–5.
4. Balogh K, Schwarz K. [Radiotherapy of neoplasms of the external ear]. Dermatologica 1968;137(4):250–8.
5. Green R, Kopf A, Bart R. X-irradiation of basal cell epitheliomas of the eyelids and canthi. In: McCarthy WH, editor. Proceedings of the International Cancer Conference. Amsterdam: VCN Blijt Publishers; 1972. p. 333–42.
6. Bart RS, Kopf AW, Petratos MA. X-ray therapy of skin cancer: evaluation of a "standardized" method for treating basal-cell epitheliomas. Proc Natl Cancer Conf 1970;6:559–69.

7. Caccialanza M, Piccinno R, Percivalle S, et al. Radiotherapy of carcinomas of the skin overlying the cartilage of the nose: our experience in 671 lesions. J Eur Acad Dermatol Venereol 2009;23(9):1044–9.
8. Caccialanza M, Piccinno R, Moretti D, et al. Radiotherapy of carcinomas of the skin overlying the cartilage of the nose: results in 405 lesions. Eur J Dermatol 2003;13(5):462–5.
9. Caccialanza M, Piccinno R, Kolesnikova L, et al. Radiotherapy of skin carcinomas of the pinna: a study of 115 lesions in 108 patients. Int J Dermatol 2005;44(6):513–7.
10. Caccialanza M, Piccinno R, Grammatica A. Radiotherapy of recurrent basal and squamous cell skin carcinomas: a study of 249 re-treated carcinomas in 229 patients. Eur J Dermatol 2001;11(1):25–8.
11. Caccialanza M, Piccinno R, Gaiani F, et al. Relevance of dermatologic radiotherapy in the therapeutic strategy of skin epithelial neoplasms: excellent results in the treatment of lesions localized on eyelids and skin overlying the cartilage of the nose. G Ital Dermatol Venereol 2013;148(1):83–8.
12. Del Regato JA, Vuksanovic M. Radiotherapy of carcinomas of the skin overlying the cartilages of the nose and ear. Radiology 1962;79:203–8.
13. Cognetta AB, Howard BM, Heaton HP, et al. Superficial x-ray in the treatment of basal and squamous cell carcinomas: a viable option in select patients. J Am Acad Dermatol 2012;67(6):1235–41.
14. Schulte KW, Lippold A, Auras C, et al. Soft x-ray therapy for cutaneous basal cell and squamous cell carcinomas. J Am Acad Dermatol 2005;53(6):993–1001.
15. Fiebelkorn HJ, Grafe E. On the therapy of tumors of the external ear. Strahlentherapie 1960;111:525–31 [in German].
16. Lim JT. Irradiation of the pinna with superficial kilovoltage radiotherapy. Clin Oncol (R Coll Radiol) 1992;4(4):236–9.
17. Moss T, Brand W, Battifora H. Radiation oncology. 5th edition. St Louis (MO): CV Mosby Co; 1979.
18. Murphy W. X-ray therapy. In: Helm F, editor. Cancer dermatology. Philadelphia: Lea & Febiger; 1979. p. 322–4.
19. Mustafa E. Ergebnisse der Nase und der Ohrmuscheln. Strahlentherapie 1966;131:505–19.
20. Panizzon RG. Die Strahlentherapie des Basalioms. In: Eichmann E, Schnyder U, editors. Das Basaliom: Der haufigste Tumor der Haut. Berlin: Springer-Verlag; 1980. p. 103–12.
21. Parker RG, Wildermuth O. Radiation therapy of lesions overlying cartilage. I. Carcinoma of the pinna. Cancer 1962;15:57–65.
22. Storck H, Ott F, Schwartz K. Haut. In: Zuppinger A, Krowski E, editors. Handbuch der Medizinischen Radiologie. Heidelberg (Germany): Springer-Verlag; 1972. p. 17–160.
23. Wiskemann A, Lippert H, Lotz G. Rontgentherapie der Basaliome, spinozellularen Karzinome und Keratoakanthome. In: Braun-Falco O, Marghescu S, editors. Fortschritte der Praktischen Dermatologies und Venerologie. Berlin: Springer-Verlag; 1976. p. 63–8.
24. Fitzpatrick PJ, Thompson GA, Easterbrook WM, et al. Basal and squamous cell carcinoma of the eyelids and their treatment by radiotherapy. Int J Radiat Oncol Biol Phys 1984;10(4):449–54.
25. Fitzpatrick PJ, Jamieson DM, Thompson GA, et al. Tumors of the eyelids and their treatment by radiotherapy. Radiology 1972;104(3):661–5.
26. Fitzpatrick PJ, Allt WE, Thompson GA. Cancer of the eyelids: their treatment by radiotherapy. Can Med Assoc J 1972;106(11):1215–1216 passim.
27. Gladstein AH. Efficacy, simplicity, and safety of X-ray therapy of basal-cell carcinomas on periocular skin. J Dermatol Surg Oncol 1978;4(8):586–93.
28. Petrovich Z, Parker RG, Luxton G, et al. Carcinoma of the lip and selected sites of head and neck skin. A clinical study of 896 patients. Radiother Oncol 1987;8(1):11–7.
29. Petrovich Z, Kuisk H, Tobochnik N, et al. Carcinoma of the lip. Arch Otolaryngol 1979;105(4):187–91.
30. Petrovich Z, Kuisk H, Langholz B, et al. Treatment results and patterns of failure in 646 patients with carcinoma of the eyelids, pinna, and nose. Am J Surg 1987;154(4):447–50.
31. Szabo P. Clinical picture and roentgen therapy of lip carcinomas. Hautarzt 1975;26(10):524–8 [in German].
32. Landthaler M, Lukacs S, Braun-Falco O, et al. Soft radiotherapy of lip cancer. Hautarzt 1981;32(2):80–3 [in German].
33. von Essen C. Roentgen therapy of skin and lip carcinoma: factors influencing success and failure. Am J Roentgenol 1960;83:556–70.
34. Traenkle HL, Stoll HL Jr, Lonkar A. Results of roentgen therapy of carcinoma of the lip. Arch Dermatol 1962;85:488–9.
35. Shore RE, Moseson M, Harley N, et al. Tumors and other diseases following childhood x-ray treatment for ringworm of the scalp (Tinea capitis). Health Phys 2003;85(4):404–8.
36. Shore RE, Albert RE, Reed M, et al. Skin cancer incidence among children irradiated for ringworm of the scalp. Radiat Res 1984;100(1):192–204.
37. Albert RE. Carcinogenic effects of radiation on the human skin. In: Upton AC, Burns FJ, Shore RE, editors. Radiation carcinogenesis. New York: Elsevier; 1986. p. 335–45.
38. Shore RE. Radiation-induced skin cancer in humans. Med Pediatr Oncol 2001;36(5):549–54.
39. Martin H, Strong E, Spiro RH. Radiation-induced skin cancer of the head and neck. Cancer 1970;25(1):61–71.

40. Karagas MR, McDonald JA, Greenberg ER, et al. Risk of basal cell and squamous cell skin cancers after ionizing radiation therapy. For The Skin Cancer Prevention Study Group. J Natl Cancer Inst 1996;88(24):1848–53.

41. Wilder RB, Kittelson JM, Shimm DS. Basal cell carcinoma treated with radiation therapy. Cancer 1991;68(10):2134–7.

42. Rowe DE, Carroll RJ, Day CL Jr. Long-term recurrence rates in previously untreated (primary) basal cell carcinoma: implications for patient follow-up. J Dermatol Surg Oncol 1989;15(3):315–28.

43. Rowe DE, Carroll RJ, Day CL Jr. Prognostic factors for local recurrence, metastasis, and survival rates in squamous cell carcinoma of the skin, ear, and lip. Implications for treatment modality selection. J Am Acad Dermatol 1992;26(6):976–90.

44. Goldschmidt H, Sherwin WK. Office radiotherapy of cutaneous carcinomas. II. Indications in specific anatomic regions. J Dermatol Surg Oncol 1983; 9(1):47–76.

45. Hernandez-Machin B, Borrego L, Gil-Garcia M, et al. Office-based radiation therapy for cutaneous carcinoma: evaluation of 710 treatments. Int J Dermatol 2007;46(5):453–9.

46. Bart RS, Kopf AW, Gladstein AH. Treatment of morphea-type basal cell carcinomas with radiation therapy. Arch Dermatol 1977;113(6):783–6.

47. Oken MM, Creech RH, Tormey DC, et al. Toxicity and response criteria of the Eastern Cooperative Oncology Group. Am J Clin Oncol 1982;5(6):649–55.

48. National Comprehensive Cancer Network (NCCN). NCCN Guidelines Version 1. Basal Cell Skin Cancer. 2015. Available at: www.nccn.org/professionals/physician_gls/pdf/nmsc.pdf. Accessed June 22, 2015.

49. National Comprehensive Cancer Network (NCCN). NCCN Guidelines Version 1. Squamous Cell Skin Cancer. 2015. Available at: www.nccn.org/professionals/physician_gls/pdf/squamous.pdf. Accessed June 22, 2015.

50. Goldschmidt H, Breneman JC, Breneman DL. Ionizing radiation therapy in dermatology. J Am Acad Dermatol 1994;30(2 Pt 1):157–82 [quiz: 183–6].

51. Erfurt-Berge C, Bauerschmitz J. Malignant tumours arising in chronic leg ulcers: three cases and a review of the literature. J Wound Care 2011;20(8): 396–400.

52. Mendenhall WM, Amdur RJ, Hinerman RW, et al. Radiotherapy for cutaneous squamous and basal cell carcinomas of the head and neck. Laryngoscope 2009;119(10):1994–9.

53. Mendenhall WM, Parsons JT, Mendenhall NP, et al. T2-T4 carcinoma of the skin of the head and neck treated with radical irradiation. Int J Radiat Oncol Biol Phys 1987;13(7):975–81.

54. Friedman DL, Whitton J, Leisenring W, et al. Subsequent neoplasms in 5-year survivors of childhood cancer: the Childhood Cancer Survivor Study. J Natl Cancer Inst 2010;102(14):1083–95.

55. Newhauser WD, Durante M. Assessing the risk of second malignancies after modern radiotherapy. Nat Rev Cancer 2011;11(6):438–48.

56. Gatti RA. The inherited basis of human radiosensitivity. Acta Oncol 2001;40(6):702–11.

57. Kleinerman RA. Radiation-sensitive genetically susceptible pediatric sub-populations. Pediatr Radiol 2009;39(Suppl 1):S27–31.

58. Jung EG. Xeroderma pigmentosum: heterogeneous syndrome and model for UV carcinogenesis. Bull Cancer 1978;65(3):315–21.

59. Gatti RA. Candidates for the molecular defect in ataxia telangiectasia. Adv Neurol 1993;61: 127–32.

60. Genetic susceptibility to cancer. ICRP publication 79. Approved by the Commission in May 1997. International Commission on Radiological Protection. Ann ICRP 1998;28(1–2):1–157.

61. Taylor AM, Harnden DG, Arlett CF, et al. Ataxia telangiectasia: a human mutation with abnormal radiation sensitivity. Nature 1975;258(5534):427–9.

62. Alter BP. Radiosensitivity in Fanconi's anemia patients. Radiother Oncol 2002;62(3):345–7.

63. Hisada M, Garber JE, Fung CY, et al. Multiple primary cancers in families with Li-Fraumeni syndrome. J Natl Cancer Inst 1998;90(8):606–11.

64. Churchill-Davidson I, Johnson E. Rodent ulcers: an analysis of 711 lesions treated by radiotherapy. Br Med J 1954;1(4877):1465–8.

65. Goldschmidt H, Sherwin WK. Office radiotherapy of cutaneous carcinomas. I. Radiation techniques, dose schedules, and radiation protection. J Dermatol Surg Oncol 1983;9(1):31–46.

66. Shack RB. Management of radiation ulcers. South Med J 1982;75(12):1462–6.

67. Goldschmidt H, Panizzon RG, editors. Modern dermatologic radiation therapy. New York: Springer-Verlag; 1991.

68. Huget-Debois H, Debois JM. Skin epithelioma of trunk and limbs. Experience with radiotherapy in 126 patients. J Belge Radiol 1991;74(2):97–103 [in Dutch].

69. de Launey JW, MacKenzie-Wood AR. Office radiotherapy in dermatology: a contemporary perspective. Australas J Dermatol 1996;37(2):71–7 [quiz: 78–9].

70. Goldschmidt H. Ionizing radiation therapy in dermatology. Current use in the United States and Canada. Arch Dermatol 1975;111(11): 1511–7.

71. Andrews GC, Domonkos AN, Hurlbut WB. Roentgen irradiation in the treatment of epithelioma. J Am Med Assoc 1954;154(1):21–2.

72. Schirren CG. The significance of soft radiation for the dermatological radiotherapy. Arch Klin Exp Dermatol 1955;199(3):228–68 [in German].

73. Renfer H. Treatment of skin tumors in the medial canthus with a special reference to the function of the lacrimal ducts. Strahlentherapie 1956;99(3): 345–53 [in German].

74. Schirren CG. A soft x-ray tube with a voltage range from 10 to 100 kV; need of soft x-ray instruments up to 100 kV for the performance of an adequate radiotherapy. Hautarzt 1956;7(1):32–6 [in German].

75. Ebbehoj E. Bucky-rays and other ultrasoft x-rays. Acta Derm Venereol 1952;32(2):117–30.

76. Jennings WA. A survey of depth dose data for X rays from 6 to 75kVp; half value layers from 0.01 to 1.0 MM AL. Br J Radiol 1953;26(309): 481–7.

77. Reisner A. Hauterythem und Röntgenstrahlung. Erg Med Strahlenforsch 1933;6:1–60.

78. Miescher G. Tierexperimentelle Untersuchungen über den Einfluss der Fraktionierung auf den Spä-teffekt. Acta Radiol 1935;16:25–38.

79. Strandquist M. A study of the cumulative effects of fractionated X-ray treatment based on the experi-ence gained at radiumhemmet with the treatment of 280 cases of carcinoma of the skin and lip. Acta Radiol 1944;55(Suppl):300–4.

80. Strandqvist M. Studien uber die kumulative Wir-kung der Rontgenstrahlen bei Fraktionierung. Acta Radiol 1944;(Suppl 55):1–300.

81. Andrews GC. Contact roentgen therapy. Arch Derm Syphilol 1948;58(2):118–27.

82. MacKee GM. X-rays and radium in the treatment of dis-eases of the skin. Philadelphia: Lea & Febiger; 1921.

83. Goldschmidt H. Dermatologic radiotherapy 1981. Arch Dermatol 1981;117(11):685–8.

84. Stoll HL Jr, Milgrom H, Traenkle HL. Results of roentgen therapy of carcinoma of the nose. Arch Dermatol 1964;90:577–80.

85. Jolly HW Jr. Superficial x-ray therapy in derma-tology–1978. Int J Dermatol 1978;17(9):691–7.

86. Nevrkla E, Newton KA. A survey of the treatment of 200 cases of basal cell carcinoma (1959-1966 in-clusive). Br J Dermatol 1974;91(4):429–33.

87. Kohlsat H, Schirren C. Die Untersuchungen von Niels Stensen uber die Haut. Versuch einer kriti-schen Betrachtung. Centaurus 1970;15:51–71.

88. Schirren CG. Rontgentherapie gutartiger und bo-sartiger Geshwulste der Haut. In: Jadassohn J, editor. Handbuch der Haut-und Geschlecht-skrankheiten, vol. 2. Berlin: Springer-Verlag; 1959. p. 289–463.

89. Schirren CG. On the current status of radiotherapy of skin cancers. Munch Med Wochenschr 1959; 101:1269–74 [in German].

90. Schirren CG. On the choice of adequate radiation qualities in roentgen therapy of skin diseases. Strahlentherapie 1959;(Suppl 43):291–303 [in German].

91. Wilder RB, Shimm DS, Kittelson JM, et al. Recur-rent basal cell carcinoma treated with radiation therapy. Arch Dermatol 1991;127(11):1668–72.

92. Chahbazian CM, Brown GS. Radiation therapy for carcinoma of the skin of the face and neck. Special considerations. JAMA 1980;244(10):1135–7.

93. Del Regato J, Spjut H. Ackerman and Del Regato's cancer: diagnosis, treatment, and prognosis. St Louis (MO): CV Mosby Co; 1977.

94. Fischbach AJ, Sause WT, Plenk HP. Radiation therapy for skin cancer. West J Med 1980; 133(5):379–82.

95. Lederman M. Radiation treatment of cancer of the eyelids. Br J Ophthalmol 1976;60(12):794–805.

96. Robins P, Bennett R. Current concepts in the man-agement of skin cancer. New York: CLINICOM; 1979.

97. Rubisz-Brzezinska J, Musialowicz D, Zebracka T. Treatment of basal cell epitheliomas. Dermatol Digest 1976;9:10–5.

98. Tsao MN, Tsang RW, Liu FF, et al. Radiotherapy man-agement for squamous cell carcinoma of the nasal skin: the Princess Margaret Hospital experience. Int J Radiat Oncol Biol Phys 2002;52(4):973–9.

99. Ashby MA, Smith J, Ainslie J, et al. Treatment of nonmelanoma skin cancer at a large Australian center. Cancer 1989;63(9):1863–71.

100. Caccialanza M, Piccinno R, Beretta M, et al. Re-sults and side effects of dermatologic radio-therapy: a retrospective study of irradiated cutaneous epithelial neoplasms. J Am Acad Der-matol 1999;41(4):589–94.

101. Chan S, Dhadda AS, Swindell R. Single fraction radiotherapy for small superficial carcinoma of the skin. Clin Oncol (R Coll Radiol) 2007;19(4):256–9.

102. Hliniak A, Maciejewski B, Trott KR. The influence of the number of fractions, overall treatment time and field size on the local control of cancer of the skin. Br J Radiol 1983;56(668):596–8.

103. Locke J, Karimpour S, Young G, et al. Radio-therapy for epithelial skin cancer. Int J Radiat Oncol Biol Phys 2001;51(3):748–55.

104. Morozov AI, Barkanov AI, Melenchuk IP, et al. Treatment of skin cancer (based on data from Mos-cow Region cancer institutes). Vopr Onkol 1976; 22(8):66–70 [in Russian].

105. Silverman MK, Kopf AW, Grin CM, et al. Recur-rence rates of treated basal cell carcinomas. Part 1: Overview. J Dermatol Surg Oncol 1991;17(9): 713–8.

106. Szabo P. Clinical picture and radiotherapy of scalp carcinomas. Z Hautkr 1978;53(13):449–52 [in German].

107. Scholefield RE. Treatment of Lupus by the X Rays. Br Med J 1900;1(2053):1083, 1082.1.

108. Pugh JW. Four Cases of rodent ulcer treated by X Rays. Br Med J 1902;1(2154):882–3.

109. Freund L. Elements of general radio-therapy for practitioners. New York, NY: Rebman; 1904.

110. Belot J. Radiotherapy in skin disease. London: Rebman; 1905.

111. Cognetta AB, Mendenhall WM, editors. Radiation therapy for skin cancer. New York: Springer; 2013.

112. Cipollaro AC, MacKee GM, Crossland PM. X rays and radium in the treatment of diseases of the skin. Philadelphia: Lea & Febiger; 1967.

113. Panizzon RG, Cooper JS, editors. Radiation treatment and radiation reactions in dermatology. Berlin, Heidelberg: Springer-Verlag; 2004.

114. Jansen GT. Treatment of basal cell epitheliomas and actinic keratoses. JAMA 1976;235(11):1152–4.

115. Traenkle HL. Management of skin cancer: basal cell epithelioma. Roentgen therapy. N Y State J Med 1968;68(7):863–5.

116. Ellis F. Dose, time and fractionation: a clinical hypothesis. Clin Radiol 1969;20(1):1–7.

117. Orton CG, Ellis F. A simplification in the use of the NSD concept in practical radiotherapy. Br J Radiol 1973;46(547):529–37.

118. Storck H. Radiotherapy of cutaneous cancers and some other malignancies. J Dermatol Surg Oncol 1978;4(8):573–84.

119. Landthaler M, Braun-Falco O. Use of the TDF factor in soft roentgen radiotherapy. Hautarzt 1989;40(12):774–7 [in German].

120. Landthaler M, Braun-Falco O. Application of TDF-factor in soft x-ray therapy. In: Orfanos CE, Stadler R, Gollnick H, editors. Proceedings of the 17th World Congress of Dermatology. Berlin, Germany: Springer-Verlag; 1988. p. 928–30.

121. Bahmer FA. Practical use of the TDF factor in radiotherapy of basalioma and squamous cell carcinoma. Hautarzt 1992;43(10):625–8 [in German].

122. Goldschmidt H. Dermatologic radiotherapy: selection of radiation qualities and treatment techniques. Int J Dermatol 1976;15(3):171–81.

123. Goldschmidt H. Radiotherapy of skin cancer: modern indications and techniques. Cutis 1976;17(2):253–61.

124. Harley NH, Kolber AB, Altman SM, et al. Determination of half-dose depth in skin for soft x-rays. J Am Acad Dermatol 1982;7(3):328–32.

125. Levy A, Stasko T. Mohs surgery. In: Alam M, editor. Evidence-based procedural dermatology. New York: Springer; 2012. p. 1–29.

126. Smeets NW, Krekels GA, Ostertag JU, et al. Surgical excision vs Mohs' micrographic surgery for basal-cell carcinoma of the face: randomised controlled trial. Lancet 2004;364(9447):1766–72.

127. Mosterd K, Krekels GA, Nieman FH, et al. Surgical excision versus Mohs' micrographic surgery for primary and recurrent basal-cell carcinoma of the face: a prospective randomised controlled trial with 5-years' follow-up. Lancet Oncol 2008;9(12):1149–56.

128. Silverman MK, Kopf AW, Gladstein AH, et al. Recurrence rates of treated basal cell carcinomas. Part 4: X-ray therapy. J Dermatol Surg Oncol 1992;18(7):549–54.

129. Ehring F, Gattwinkel U. Radiotherapy of upper lip basalioma. Hautarzt 1974;25(8):368–72 [in German].

130. Veness MJ, Harris D. Role of radiotherapy in the management of organ transplant recipients diagnosed with non-melanoma skin cancers. Australas Radiol 2007;51(1):12–20.

131. Silva JJ, Tsang RW, Panzarella T, et al. Results of radiotherapy for epithelial skin cancer of the pinna: the Princess Margaret Hospital experience, 1982-1993. Int J Radiat Oncol Biol Phys 2000;47(2):451–9.

132. Lukas VanderSpek LA, Pond GR, Wells W, et al. Radiation therapy for Bowen's disease of the skin. Int J Radiat Oncol Biol Phys 2005;63(2):505–10.

133. Croce O, Hachem S, Franchisseur E, et al. Jean-MarcBordy. Contact radiotherapy using a 50 kV X-ray system: evaluation of relative dose distribution with the Monte Carlo code PENELOPE and comparison with measurements. Radiat Phys Chem 2012;81(6):609–17.

134. Rogers HW, Coldiron BM. A relative value unit-based cost comparison of treatment modalities for nonmelanoma skin cancer: effect of the loss of the Mohs multiple surgery reduction exemption. J Am Acad Dermatol 2009;61(1):96–103.

135. Alam M, Berg D, Bhatia A, et al. Association between number of stages in Mohs micrographic surgery and surgeon-, patient-, and tumor-specific features: a cross-sectional study of practice patterns of 20 early- and mid-career Mohs surgeons. Dermatol Surg 2010;36(12):1915–20.

136. Bhatnagar A, Loper A. The initial experience of electronic brachytherapy for the treatment of nonmelanoma skin cancer. Radiat Oncol 2010;5:87.

137. Solan JM, Brady LW. Skin cancer. In: Halperin EC, Perez CA, Brady LW, editors. Principles and practice of radiation oncology. 5th edition. Philadelphia: Lippincott Williams & Wilkins; 2008. p. 690–700.

138. Accreditation Council for Graduate Medical Education (ACGME). ACGME Program Requirements for Graduate Medical Education in Dermatology. 2014.

139. Nair R, Aggarwal R, Khanna D. Methods of formal consensus in classification/diagnostic criteria and guideline development. Semin Arthritis Rheum 2011;41(2):95–105.

140. Shekelle PG, Ortiz E, Rhodes S, et al. Validity of the Agency for Healthcare Research and Quality clinical practice guidelines: how quickly do guidelines become outdated? JAMA 2001;286(12):1461–7.

141. Silverman MK, Kopf AW, Grin CM, et al. Recurrence rates of treated basal cell carcinomas. Part 2: curettage-electrodesiccation. J Dermatol Surg Oncol 1991;17(9):720–6.

142. Maloney M, Miller S. Aggressive vs nonaggressive subtypes (basal cell carcinoma). In: Miller S, Maloney M, editors. Cutaneous oncology pathophysiology, diagnosis, and management. Malden (MA): Blackwell Science; 1998. p. 494–5.

143. Salasche S. Features associated with recurrence (squamous cell carcinoma). In: Miller CJ, Maloney ME, editors. Cutaneous oncology pathophysiology, diagnosis, and management. Malden (MA): Blackwell Science; 1998. p. 494–9.

144. Boeta-Angeles L, Bennett R. Features associated with recurrence (basal cell carcinoma). In: Miller S, Maloney ME, editors. Cutaneous oncology pathophysiology, diagnosis, and management. Malden (MA): Blackwell Science; 1998. p. 500–5.

145. Haas A. Features associated with metastasis (squamous cell carcinoma). In: Miller S, Maloney ME, editors. Cutaneous oncology pathophysiology, diagnosis, and management. Malden (MA): Blackwell Sciences; 1998. p. 500–5.

146. Randle HW. Basal cell carcinoma. Identification and treatment of the high-risk patient. Dermatol Surg 1996;22(3):255–61.

147. Rieger KE, Linos E, Egbert BM, et al. Recurrence rates associated with incompletely excised low-risk nonmelanoma skin cancer. J Cutan Pathol 2010;37(1):59–67.

148. Ulrich C, Kanitakis J, Stockfleth E, et al. Skin cancer in organ transplant recipients–where do we stand today? Am J Transplant 2008;8(11):2192–8.

149. Patel RV, Clark LN, Lebwohl M, et al. Treatments for psoriasis and the risk of malignancy. J Am Acad Dermatol 2009;60(6):1001–17.

150. Euvrard S, Kanitakis J, Claudy A. Skin cancers after organ transplantation. N Engl J Med 2003;348(17):1681–91.

151. Lott DG, Manz R, Koch C, et al. Aggressive behavior of nonmelanotic skin cancers in solid organ transplant recipients. Transplantation 2010;90(6):683–7.

152. Brodland D. Features associated with metastasis (basal cell carcinoma). In: Miller S, Maloney M, editors. Cutaneous oncology pathophysiology, diagnosis, and management. Malden (MA): Blackwell Science; 1998. p. 657–63.

153. Edwards MJ, Hirsch RM, Broadwater JR, et al. Squamous cell carcinoma arising in previously burned or irradiated skin. Arch Surg 1989;124(1):115–7.

154. Mendenhall WM, Ferlito A, Takes RP, et al. Cutaneous head and neck basal and squamous cell carcinomas with perineural invasion. Oral Oncol 2012;48(10):918–22.

155. Kyrgidis A, Tzellos TG, Kechagias N, et al. Cutaneous squamous cell carcinoma (SCC) of the head and neck: risk factors of overall and recurrence-free survival. Eur J Cancer 2010;46(9):1563–72.

156. Galloway TJ, Morris CG, Mancuso AA, et al. Impact of radiographic findings on prognosis for skin carcinoma with clinical perineural invasion. Cancer 2005;103(6):1254–7.

157. Eaglstein WH. Evidence-based medicine, the research-practice gap, and biases in medical and surgical decision making in dermatology. Arch Dermatol 2010;146(10):1161–4.

158. Kingery FA. Radiation therapy in dermatologic training centers. J Am Acad Dermatol 1986;14(6):1108–10.

159. Schalock PC, Carter J, Zug KA. Use of ionizing radiation in dermatologic training centers. J Am Acad Dermatol 2006;55(5):912–3.

Practice and Educational Gaps in Surgery for Skin Cancer

Murad Alam, MD, MSCI, MBA[a,b,c,]*, Abigail Waldman, MD[a],
Ian A. Maher, MD[d]

KEYWORDS

- Practice gaps • Educational gaps • Skin cancer • Surgical treatment

KEY POINTS

- This article defines the current practice in surgical treatment of skin cancers by dermatologists, gaps in practice, and mechanisms to improve current surgical practice.
- Although treatment of more common nonmelanoma skin cancers is standardized, differential access and availability of specialty services and a lack of guidelines for several rare skin cancers can result in inconsistent treatment.
- Affiliations or referral to academic or larger medical centers for the treatment of complex skin cancers and the development of best practice guidelines for aggressive or rare tumors may remedy the shortcomings in current practice.
- Additionally, education in dermatologic surgery and management of skin cancer is improved by exposing residents to more cases of complex tumor management during training, including simulation of complex tumor cases, continuity clinics, and encouraging postresidency training when appropriate.

Surgery for skin cancer is a major part of clinical dermatology, and the largest single component of dermatologic surgery practice. In general, residency training in dermatology provides comprehensive training in the theory and practice of skin cancer surgery. Practicing dermatologists are similarly expert in this area, and frequently assist other medical and surgical services by managing and coordinating the care of patients with skin cancer. Even so, there are some minor gaps in training and practice that bear scrutiny and are amenable to rectification.

PRACTICE GAPS IN CLINICAL DERMATOLOGY PRACTICE

Best Practices

Best practices for surgery for skin cancer vary based on the histologic type of cancer, clinical features of the cancer, and patient-specific factors. Still, there are some common elements in appropriate care (**Box 1**).

Before surgery, key data pertaining to the case are obtained, collated, and reviewed. Relevant information includes the biopsy reports and any other laboratory tests or diagnostic imaging.

Financial Disclosures and Conflicts of Interest: None.

Funding Support: This publication was supported by Merz Center for Quality and Outcomes Research in Dermatologic Surgery and the IMPROVED (Measurement of Priority Outcome Variables in Dermatologic Surgery) group.

[a] Department of Dermatology, Feinberg School of Medicine, Northwestern University, 676 North St. Clair Street, Suite 1600, Chicago, IL 60611, USA; [b] Department of Otolaryngology, Feinberg School of Medicine, Northwestern University, 676 North St. Clair Street, Suite 1600, Chicago, IL 60611, USA; [c] Department of Surgery, Feinberg School of Medicine, Northwestern University, 676 North St. Clair Street, Suite 1600, Chicago, IL 60611, USA; [d] Department of Dermatology, Saint Louis University, 1755 South Grand Blvd., St Louis, MO 63104, USA

* Corresponding author. Department of Dermatology, 676 North St. Clair Street, Suite 1600, Chicago, IL 60611.

E-mail address: m-alam@northwestern.edu

Dermatol Clin 34 (2016) 335–339
http://dx.doi.org/10.1016/j.det.2016.02.012

> **Box 1**
> **Surgery of the skin: practice gaps**
>
> *Best Practice*
>
> - Before surgery, key data pertaining to the case are obtained, collated, and reviewed. Additional diagnostic tests or confirmatory reads of existing raw data by additional specialized authorities (eg, dermatopathology, radiology) may be required.
>
> - Staging of the tumor, if appropriate, is performed in accordance with American Joint Committee on Cancer criteria and other clarifying literature. Reference to clinical practice guidelines, including those promulgated by the National Comprehensive Cancer Network and relevant specialty societies (eg, American Academy of Dermatology, American Society for Dermatologic Surgery), is considered.
>
> - Appropriate referral when medically necessary.
>
> - Appropriate follow-up care to monitor for recurrence or new primary tumors.
>
> *How Current Practices Differ from Best Practice*
>
> - Differential access and availability of other specialty services that may be required to manage complex or aggressive skin cancers.
>
> - No available guidelines of care for several rare skin cancers resulting in inconsistent treatments across centers.
>
> *Barriers to Best Practice Implementation*
>
> - Atomized nature of dermatology practice that may not be in proximity to referral centers or other specialists' offices.
>
> - Barriers to development of more detailed practice guidelines and guidelines for the management of rare circumstances include limitations in the medical evidence.
>
> *Strategies to Overcome Barriers*
>
> - Affiliations with local academic medical centers or multispecialty practices may help overcome this barrier. Provisions for such alliances will likely need to overcome financial and regulatory disincentives to collaboration.
>
> - Development of large prospective databases documenting patient care parameters by the American Academy of Dermatology and the American College of Mohs Surgery Formation of consensus groups to develop practice guidelines for management of aggressive or rare skin tumors.

Unusual findings on diagnostic tests may suggest the need for additional tests, or confirmatory reads of existing raw data by additional specialized authorities (eg, dermatopathology, radiology). Staging of the tumor, if appropriate, is performed in accordance with American Joint Committee on Cancer criteria and other clarifying literature. Reference to clinical practice guidelines, including those promulgated by the National Comprehensive Cancer Network and relevant specialty societies (eg, American Academy of Dermatology, American Society for Dermatologic Surgery), is considered. Aspects of care where guidance is unavailable or ambiguous can be determined by consideration of patient-specific factors; discussion with the patient, patient's family, and other members of the medical team; and if appropriate, via a formal ethics board or tumor board consultation. When care in addition to dermatologic surgery may be necessary, additional referrals may be made to other specialists (eg, surgical oncology, plastic surgery, head and neck surgery,

urogynecological surgery, transplant medicine or surgery, medical oncology, and radiation oncology). After surgery, appropriate follow-up care to monitor for recurrence or new primary tumors is implemented. Dysfunction or disfigurement resulting from prior surgeries is managed (eg, treatment of hypertrophic or symptomatic scars, treatment of functional asymmetry).

Current Practice

Current practice is variable. Treatment of primary and recurrent basal cell carcinomas and squamous cell carcinomas of small to moderate size and low to moderate risk is consistent at many centers. Higher risk lesions are addressed by Mohs surgery, with lower risk tumors treated by excision, electrodessication and curettage, or other methods. In general, National Comprehensive Cancer Network guidelines are observed.

Treatment of higher risk tumors, including locally advanced or metastatic basal cell carcinoma; high-risk, locally advanced, or metastatic cutaneous squamous cell carcinoma; Merkel cell carcinoma; melanoma; and rare nonmelanoma skin cancers is less consistent across centers. The rates at which other services are consulted and interdisciplinary plans are initiated regarding the management of higher risk tumors range from low to high. Rates of adjuvant treatment are also different. Some centers are more prepared to provide surgical treatment of higher risk skin cancers, and other centers are more likely to refer these to other dermatologic surgery centers.

Gaps and their Classification

Current gaps include differential access and availability of other specialty services that may be required to manage complex or aggressive skin cancers. Additionally, there are no guidelines of care for several rare nonmelanoma skin cancers because of the extreme rarity of these. Emerging useful treatment options, such as 100% margin controlled excision for melanoma-in-situ of the head and neck, are variably used. For some cancers, there are no well-established follow-up treatment plans, including a lack of recommendations regarding future surveillance and testing.

The limited degree of interdisciplinary care transcends the range of categories from knowledge, to skill, to attitude, to specific practices. Practitioners may not be aware of usual and customary practices at major treatment centers, or recommended practices in recent clinical guidelines. For example, the use of sentinel lymph node biopsy and PET/computed tomography for Merkel cell carcinoma, both of which have been shown strong prognostic value for Merkel cell carcinoma, is highly variable.[1,2] In terms of skill and attitude, practitioners may have a preference for managing even complex tumors entirely in-house, or may not have active referral or consulting relationships with other specialists. The gaps pertaining to limitations or omissions in current guidelines, or the absence of practice guidelines for certain tumor types, are primarily gaps in knowledge.

Barriers and How They May Be Overcome

Principal barriers include the atomized nature of dermatology practice, where many practitioners practice in solo or small specialty-specific groups that are not in physical proximity to referral centers or other specialists' offices. The outstanding, convenient, and patient-friendly personalized service that dermatologists can offer patients in their private offices paradoxically limits the ease of collaboratively managing with other specialists

the few patients who may benefit from interdisciplinary care. Affiliations with local academic medical centers or multispecialty practices may help overcome this barrier. Provisions for such alliances will likely need to overcome financial and regulatory disincentives to collaboration.

Barriers to development of more detailed practice guidelines and guidelines for the management of rare circumstances include limitations in the medical evidence. Development of large prospective databases documenting patient care parameters by the American Academy of Dermatology and the American College of Mohs Surgery will result in copious data on management of aggressive and rare skin cancers. These outcomes data can then be used by consensus groups to develop preliminary practice guidelines for these circumstances. Several years of data collection will likely be required before the data are sifted and analyzed in this manner.

As these and other new data are developed they need to be efficiently and rapidly disseminated to providers. Internet-based educational resources provide a ready means to effectively communicate information and have shown to be effective modifiers of physician practice.[3] As medical practice becomes ever more complex, these types of self-paced "on-demand" educational interventions may prove to have a higher impact than traditional means of distributing medical knowledge (such as journals or conventions.) An additional advantage of the World Wide Web is the ability to connect the aforementioned atomized dermatology providers and their patients with expertise that may be otherwise geographically remote and unavailable to them.

EDUCATIONAL GAPS IN DERMATOLOGY RESIDENCY EDUCATION
Best Practices and Current Practices

Best practices and current practices in residency training environments are similar to those in general clinical practice, with some differences. Residency training programs are usually situated in academic medical centers, where adherence to clinical practice guidelines and interdisciplinary skin cancer care may be more common. For instance, some residents participate in tumor boards. Moreover, some academic medical centers staff specialized dermatology clinics for management of aggressive skin cancers, such as transplant-associated squamous cell carcinoma, Merkel cell carcinoma, or melanoma. Residents are trained in patient selection, preoperative preparation, surgical technique, reconstruction of defects, postoperative care, and management of adverse events. The quantity of relevant training is variable based on time allocation for such at different residency programs.

Additionally, how learners' performance is assessed is variable. Although some objective assessment tools have been developed for a few basic procedures, their use is far from universal.[4] Given the relative dearth of objective assessment, those few learners who struggle with surgical skills and principles may not be identified for additional educational interventions while in residency (**Box 2**).

Gaps and Their Classification

Management of aggressive and complex skin cancers is an area where dermatology residents may have limited expertise. Residents may lack extensive experience in the indications that might benefit from multidisciplinary care, including adjuvant diagnostic tests, such as imaging, or adjuvant therapy, such as radiation or oral chemoprevention. Residents at different centers may also have more or less training in specific techniques of skin cancer removal; in general, training is more rudimentary

in advanced techniques, such as Mohs surgery. Training may also be deficient in the area of management of adverse events, because of their infrequency in dermatologic surgery. Primarily, training gaps are in knowledge and skill.

Barriers and How They May Be Overcome

A major obstacle to educating dermatology residents regarding surgical treatment of skin cancer is the limited time available for surgical dermatology during the 3 years of training. This inhibits the conveyance of necessary knowledge, and even more, the development of visuospatial and hand skills that require sustained, repeated practice. Management of aggressive and complex skin requires continuity over several months or years, and residents may be rotated off services on a monthly basis. Because postoperative adverse events occur after fewer than 1% of skin cancer surgeries, their relative infrequency limits the number of cases from which residents can learn. Reconstruction after cancer surgery is a vast area that comprises many types of linear repairs, flaps, and grafts, and requires seeing and

---

Box 2
Surgery of skin: educational gaps

Best Practice

- Training programs are usually situated in academic medical centers, where adherence to clinical practice guidelines and interdisciplinary skin cancer care may be more common, often with access to specialized dermatology clinics for management of aggressive skin cancers.
- Residents are trained in patient selection, preoperative preparation, surgical technique, reconstruction of defects, postoperative care, and management of adverse events.

How Current Practices Differ from Best Practice

- Management of aggressive and complex skin cancers is an area where dermatology residents may have limited expertise.
- Training in specific techniques of skin cancer removal varies among training programs and may be deficient in procedures, such as Mohs surgery, or management of adverse events.

Barriers to Best Practice Implementation

- Limited time available for surgical dermatology during the 3 years of training.
- Exposure to adverse events and their management may be limited.

Strategies to Overcome Barriers

- Simulations of complex tumor cases where residents are provided with history and diagnostic information may improve knowledge and skill in this area. Attendance at tumor board.
- Continuity clinics where residents were able to follow complex tumors during the course of their residency may provide them with further insight into the time course of such tumors, and not only the physical but also the psychological impact on the patient.
- Practice performing tumor removals and reconstructions on computer models, physical surgical models, formalin-fixed cadavers, or fresh frozen cadaver heads. Classroom instruction in surgical anatomy and computer animations showing tissue movement in flaps may also accelerate learning.
- Completion of additional postresidency training.

performing many cases, which may not be available for all residents at most centers.

To overcome the time limitations of residency is challenging. Simulations of complex tumor cases, where residents are provided with history and diagnostic information and asked to develop a plan, may improve knowledge and skill in this area. Attendance at tumor board, where residents may hear complex cases discussed, may allow residents to better understand the management of complex, aggressive, and rare skin tumors. Continuity clinics where residents were able to follow complex tumors during the course of their residency may provide them with further insight into the time course of such tumors, and not only the physical but also the psychological impact on the patient. This, in turn, may help residents approach such patients in a more caring, supportive, and realistic manner. It is unlikely that even the busiest clinical skin cancer surgery services are able to provide enough cases for all residents to achieve skill proficiency in cancer removal and reconstruction. To augment the available cases, residents may perform removals and reconstructions on computer models, physical surgical models, formalin-fixed cadavers, or fresh frozen cadaver heads. Classroom instruction in surgical anatomy and computer animations showing tissue movement in flaps may also accelerate learning. Additionally electronic media provide a powerful means for disseminating information and sharing resources between training programs.[5] The pooling of resources among training programs presents an avenue for providing a more complete and consistent education to residents who do not have access to certain resources via their home training programs.[4]

One well-established means for overcoming barriers pertaining to knowledge and skill is completion of additional postresidency training. Such training most often takes the form of an Accreditation Council for Graduate Medical Education–approved fellowship in Micrographic Surgery and Dermatologic Oncology. Recently renamed, this 1-year fellowship has a primary emphasis on skin cancer removal and reconstruction, and ensures that every fellow completes at least several hundred cases independently. Fellows are also trained in collaboration with other services.

REFERENCES

1. Sadeghi R, Adinehpoor Z, Maleki M, et al. Prognostic significance of sentinel lymph node mapping in Merkel cell carcinoma: systematic review and meta-analysis of prognostic studies. Biomed Res Int 2014;2014:489536.
2. Ibrahim SF, Ahronowitz I, McCalmont TH, et al. 18F-fluorodeoxyglucose positron emission tomography-computed tomography imaging in the management of Merkel cell carcinoma: a single-institution retrospective study. Dermatol Surg 2013;39(9):1323–33.
3. Eide MJ, Asgari MM, Fletcher SW, et al, INFORMED (INternet course FOR Melanoma Early Detection) Group. Effects on skills and practice from a web-based skin cancer course for primary care providers. J Am Board Fam Med 2013;26(6):648–57.
4. Alam M, Nodzenski M, Yoo S, et al. Objective structured assessment of technical skills in elliptical excision repair of senior dermatology residents: a multirater, blinded study of operating room video recordings. JAMA Dermatol 2014; 150(6):608–12.
5. Koya KD, Bhatia KR, Hsu JT, et al. YouTube and the expanding role of videos in dermatologic surgery education. Semin Cutan Med Surg 2012;31(3):163–7.

Practice and Educational Gaps in Cosmetic Dermatologic Surgery

Abigail Waldman, MD[a], Joseph F. Sobanko, MD[b],
Murad Alam, MD, MSCI, MBA[a,c,d],*

KEYWORDS

• Practice gaps • Educational gaps • Cosmetic dermatologic surgery • Best practice

KEY POINTS

• This article identifies the current gaps in the practice of cosmetic dermatology, cosmetics education, and how to best overcome these limitations.
• First, there is a rapid development of new devices and procedures, with limited data, patient-reported outcomes, and comparative effectiveness research from which to develop best cosmetic practice.
• Unfortunately, there is limited funding available to ascertain such data.
• We suggest that there is a need for increased research and funding dedicated to these goals, improved and convenient training for staff looking to adopt new devices/procedures, and continuous evolution of databases to pool outcome data and develop outcome sets.
• Additionally, resident education can be improved by dedicated resident cosmetic clinics, didactic teaching from visiting professors, attendance of cosmetic dermatology courses and meetings, and encouraging postresidency training.

Cosmetic dermatologic surgery has been an integral part of dermatology practice for more than half a century. Procedures that have been developed by dermatologists include hair transplants, tumescent liposuction, botulinum toxin for facial rhytids, many cutaneous laser and light devices, and soft tissue augmentation injectables. In recent decades, cosmetic dermatologic surgery has evolved from a few related procedures to a major subfield of dermatology, an expansive and coherent body of knowledge that is increasingly viewed by others as part of the special expertise of dermatologists. Residency training in such procedures is increasing, and a growing fraction of the typical dermatologists' practice is devoted to cosmetic procedures. Fellowship training in cosmetic dermatologic surgery has been accredited by the American Society for Dermatologic Surgery (ASDS) since 2013. Recent research has confirmed that primary care physicians view dermatologists as the preeminent specialists for many cosmetic procedures, including neurotoxins, fillers, and lasers.[1]

Financial Disclosures and Conflicts of Interest: None.
Funding Support: This publication was supported by Merz Center for Quality and Outcomes Research in Dermatologic Surgery and the IMPROVED (Measurement of Priority Outcome Variables in Dermatologic Surgery) group.
[a] Department of Dermatology, Feinberg School of Medicine, Northwestern University, 676 North St. Clair Street, Suite 1600, Chicago, IL 60611, USA; [b] Department of Dermatology, University of Pennsylvania, 3400 Civic Center Boulevard, Philadelphia, PA 19104, USA; [c] Department of Otolaryngology, Feinberg School of Medicine, Northwestern University, 676 N. St. Clair, Suite 1600, Chicago, IL 60611, USA; [d] Department of Surgery, Feinberg School of Medicine, Northwestern University, 676 N. St. Clair, Suite 1600, Chicago, IL 60611, USA
* Corresponding author. Department of Dermatology, 676 North St. Clair Street, Suite 1600, Chicago, IL 60611.
E-mail address: m-alam@northwestern.edu

Dermatol Clin 34 (2016) 341–346
http://dx.doi.org/10.1016/j.det.2016.03.001

PRACTICE GAPS IN CLINICAL DERMATOLOGY PRACTICE
Best Practices

Best practices for cosmetic dermatologic surgery pertain to various elements of patient care: patient selection, the cosmetic consultation, development of a treatment plan, selection of procedures, performance of procedures, management of adverse events, and follow-up (**Box 1**). Cosmetic dermatologic surgery is a broad area, and individual variation is the norm. General best practices are described in this article. Practices specific to laser and light treatments, whether cosmetic or medically necessary, are reviewed elsewhere in this issue (See Murad Alam, Abigail Waldman, Keyvan Nouri, et al: Practice and Educational Gaps in Light, Laser, and Energy Treatments, in this issue).

Regarding patient selection, best practice includes avoiding procedures on patients with body dysmorphic disorder or unrealistic expectations. Psychological concerns are often integral motivators for patients seeking cosmetic procedures, so a necessary next step is a cosmetic consultation where the patient and dermatologist get to know one another; the dermatologist understands the patient's concerns, preferences, and risk threshold; and the patient comes to understand what is possible, and how much it may cost in terms of time, money, risk, and downtime. At the culmination of the cosmetic consultation, a treatment plan is developed that entails one or more procedures delivered over a defined time window to achieve specific objectives.

Cosmetic dermatologic procedures are safe outpatient procedures usually performed under local anesthesia. Best practice includes using Food and Drug Administration–approved drugs and devices, or other appropriate mechanisms, in a manner that poses minimal risk to the patient

---

Box 1
Cosmetic dermatologic surgery: practice gaps

Best Practice

- Personnel delivering procedures be well-trained in that procedure, and if not a dermatologist themselves, be supervised by a qualified dermatologist.

- Cosmetic consultation with appropriate patient selection and close follow-up.

- Trained use of Food and Drug Administration–approved drugs and devices, or other appropriate mechanisms, in a manner that poses minimal risk to the patient and is associated with a reasonable likelihood of success.

- Reference of available guidelines for care and consensus statements when available.

How Current Practices Differ from Best Practice

- Rapid rate of change within field with newer materials and advanced techniques not adopted by all practitioners.

- Cosmetic procedures may often be delegated to ancillary staff.

- Dearth of high-quality posttreatment patient-reported outcome data with few reliable standardized measurement tools to assess clinical outcomes after cosmetic procedures, limiting patient and practitioner clinical decision-making.

Barriers to Best Practice Implementation

- Need for improved, increased, and more accessible training for clinicians.

- Limited research funding, work force focused on clinical outcomes, and multicenter pooled data.

Strategies to Overcome Barriers

- Availability of convenient, practical, and concise on-line education in addition to improved in-office training of dermatologists by clinical staff employed by the manufacturer.

- Increase in research funding and fellow research commitments to improve pool of future investigators.

- Creation of on-line databases to pool data across centers (eg, Dermbase), development of core outcome sets (eg, those developed by IMPROVED group) should be continued and expanded. Once core outcome sets are implemented, patients and physicians will be better able to select procedures and products that are most suited to a particular patient's circumstances.

and is associated with a reasonable likelihood of success. Safety is particularly important given the elective nature of cosmetic procedures, but it is also crucial to convey to the patient that all risk cannot be eliminated and that serious adverse events, although unlikely, can occur in the absence of any treatment error.

Copious published literature and information about customary practice discussed at national and regional professional meetings can clarify procedure technique. Guidelines for care and consensus statements regarding best approaches to care are available for various procedures, including liposuction, fillers, neuromodulators, and lasers and energy devices. Similarly, current literature and expert groups can be consulted regarding management of any adverse events that may occur.

Cosmetic dermatologic treatments are often done in series, or may have a temporary benefit, so routine follow-up includes determining appropriate intervals for retreatment, or additional touch-ups. Best practice, as defined by such flagship professional societies as ASDS, is that any personnel delivering procedures be well-trained in that procedure, and if not a dermatologist themselves, be supervised by a qualified dermatologist.

Current Practice

Some newer materials are not used by all practitioners, and some more advanced techniques are not widely practiced. Cosmetic consultations and treatment plans may be limited by the scope of procedures offered by a particular practice or practitioner. Because of the rarity of adverse events,[2] rare adverse events may be seen more infrequently in lower volume practices, which may consequently be less experienced in their treatment. Some procedures are delivered by dermatologists, and some are delegated to ancillary staff,[3] such as mid-level nonphysician providers, trained by them and under their direct supervision. Some dermatologists are more likely to delegate procedures. State government regulation regarding scope of practice and delegation of cosmetic procedures is limited.[4] Cosmetic procedures performed by less-trained staff seem to be more likely to result in adverse outcomes and litigation.[5–7]

Gaps and Their Classification

Gaps include slow or variable adoption of novel procedures, with some practitioners more likely to add these to their clinical armamentarium. Additionally, practitioners may also vary in how many different procedures they offer. As a result, patients may be more or less able to obtain particular procedures depending on the dermatologists they select. These gaps pertain to knowledge, skill, attitude, and practice.

There is a relative dearth of high-quality post-treatment patient-reported outcome data. In particular, patient preferences and satisfaction are poorly understood in the context of cosmetic procedures. There are few reliable standardized measurement tools to assess clinical outcomes after cosmetic procedures. Comparative effectiveness research that evaluates the effectiveness, cost, longevity of effect, patient acceptance, or safety of procedures for similar indications is in its infancy. These research gaps impact the knowledge available to practicing dermatologists.

Barriers and How They May Be Overcome

Principal barriers include the rapid rate of change in cosmetic dermatologic surgery, with this inhibiting the ability of dermatologists to stay fully trained in the latest techniques. A related barrier is the medical rather than cosmetic emphasis of many dermatologists who perform some cosmetic procedures; such dermatologists may have limited time to perform cosmetic procedures and may lack the interest to add low-volume or resource-intensive techniques to their practices.

From a patient standpoint, it is difficult to ascertain which devices or procedures may be most effective, and which practice is best for their needs. Patients are bombarded with myriad advertisements and social media sites promoting cosmetic procedures and individual practitioners, and patients can struggle to determine which information sources are most credible.

From a research standpoint, a major barrier is the limited funding available. Federal grants are rare for investigations related to cosmetic procedures. Third-party payers, who do not reimburse cosmetic procedures, are unlikely to invest in clinical or comparative effectiveness research. Most relevant research is performed by drug and device companies, and is narrowly targeted to obtaining Food and Drug Administration clearance or approval. Research performed by entities with a principal financial interest in the success of the products being tested may be subject to obvious potential conflicts of interest. Manufacturers of cosmetic products prefer to avoid comparative effectiveness research that may show their products to be less effective than competitors'. In addition, cosmetic procedures are inherently difficult to compare because common treatment approaches may include several different types of procedures performed serially or in parallel over some period of time. Therefore comparing a single treatment of a particular type with a single treatment of a different type may not yield information that is clinically relevant. It may also be difficult to find investigators who are equally expert in the procedures being compared. Finally, few useful outcome measures for delineating procedure success are available. Metrics for assessing treatment success are often unreliable subjective global measures based on brief, nonvalidated patient or investigator questionnaires.

To overcome the training problem posed by rapid change and advancement in cosmetic procedures, there is a need for improved, increased, and more accessible training. Currently, training is provided mostly by product manufacturers or distributors, specialized education companies, and major professional societies. Manufacturers have detailed information about their own products, are highly incentivized to increase use, and have clinical experts on staff who are able to provide technical training in the use of their products. However, manufacturers may be less motivated to point out the limitations of their products or procedures, or to suggest alternatives that may be preferred in certain situations. On the other hand, manufacturers may be able to send trainers directly into dermatologist offices, thus conveniently educating dermatologists who do not need to take time off to travel to other venues. Manufacturers are highly motivated to provide training that minimizes the risk of adverse events, which could reflect poorly on the product. Specialized education companies may be able to provide a more balanced education than manufacturers. Professional societies can provide World Wide Web–based education or courses at national or regional meetings, they exist mostly to serve their members, and are generally not-for-profit. Training in cosmetic procedures can be improved by an increased effort by manufacturers and professional societies to provide on-line education that dermatologists can access at their convenience. This education should be practical and concise, and may make use of animations that illustrate treatment technique. Routine in-office training of dermatologists by clinical staff employed by the manufacturer would also help ensure that dermatologists are up-to-date regarding the latest products and their use.

Manufacturers may also choose to support research into medical indications for devices and drugs that already have well-established cosmetic indications. At present, given the dearth of reimbursable CPT codes for such products as lasers and injectables, and the consequent uncertain insurer reimbursement for these, manufacturers have focused primarily on the self-pay, cosmetic market. Research on medical indications for approved cosmetic products and procedures is therefore often ad hoc and unfunded, comprised of individual case reports or case series from enterprising physicians. Growth in the number and quality of medical indications may be hastened if manufacturers invest more research in this area.

The barrier posed by limited research funds is an imposing one. Comparative effectiveness research is to some extent supported by the professional societies, such as the Dermatology Foundation, the ASDS, and the American Society for Laser Medicine and Surgery. The amounts provided are modest, and could be increased significantly. Mandating more extensive research commitments by fellows in training could create an enlarged body of young, trained experts in clinical research to conduct future investigations. The creation of on-line databases to pool data across centers, as has already been initiated by some groups (eg, Dermbase), could be continued and expanded.

Core outcome sets can be developed for cosmetic procedures so that effectiveness, safety, and tolerability can be compared across studies and procedures. The IMPROVED group is currently working on such core outcome sets, which include investigator-rated outcomes and patient-reported outcomes. Once core outcome sets are implemented, patients and physicians will be better able to select procedures and products that are most suited to a particular patient's circumstances.

EDUCATIONAL GAPS IN DERMATOLOGY RESIDENCY EDUCATION
Best Practices

Best practice ensures that graduating residents become proficient in the performance of a range of cosmetic dermatologic procedures, including neuromodulator injections, soft tissue augmentation, sclerotherapy and treatment of leg veins, and scar revision (**Box 2**). Residents may also be competent in advanced procedures, such as liposuction, rhytidectomy or blepharoplasty, or endovenous laser treatment.[6]

Current Practices

Current practice is highly variable. Some residency programs ensure resident competence in all the basic cosmetic procedures listed previously, and some advanced procedures. Usually, these programs are based in dermatology departments with a large cosmetic practice staffed by

---

Box 2
Cosmetic dermatologic surgery: educational gaps

Best Practice

- Residents are proficient in a range of basic cosmetic dermatologic procedures and be familiar with more advanced procedures

How Current Practices Differ from Best Practice

- Cosmetic training is highly variable based on residency with some dermatology trainees unable to become proficient in basic cosmetic procedures

Barriers to Best Practice Implementation

- Limited time restraints during residency and a dearth of full-time cosmetic dermatology faculty in dermatology departments supporting residency programs limits resident access to appropriate training

Strategies to Overcome Barriers

- Development of resident cosmetic surgery clinics with discounted fees for volunteer patients with faculty oversight from within the institution, volunteer and private practice dermatologists
- Didactic teaching from visiting professors from other institutions and resident away rotations
- Resident encouragement to attend cosmetic dermatology courses and meetings (eg, those hosted by the American Academy of Dermatology and ASDS)
- Completion of additional postresidency training

---

one or more dedicated cosmetic dermatologists.[8,9] In some other programs, cosmetic dermatologic surgery education in residency consists of some hands-on training in injectables and possibly sclerotherapy. Some programs may also provide lectures and didactic information on indications and technique of other cosmetic procedures in which resident competence is not achieved.

Gaps and Their Classification

Some dermatology trainees may not be competent in the entire range of cosmetic dermatologic procedures by the end of residency. These are gaps in knowledge and skill.

Barriers and How They May Be Overcome

Barriers include limited time to train residents in cosmetic procedures, and a dearth of full-time cosmetic dermatology faculty in dermatology departments supporting residency programs. As of this writing, Accreditation Council for Graduate Medical Education dermatology residency requirements do not require hands-on proficiency in all cosmetic procedures. Observation of certain procedures or didactic training on particular advanced procedures is accepted in lieu of hands-on proficiency.

Time in residency is limited, so this barrier is best overcome by increasing the efficiency of training in cosmetic dermatologic surgery.

Resident cosmetic surgery clinics can be established in which faculty supervise residents, who work on cosmetic patients attracted by heavily discounted fees and willing to have hands-on treatment from residents-in-training. Such clinics can occur as frequently as one or several half days a month, thus limiting time away from other resident responsibilities. Residents can also be made in charge of recruiting patients for these clinics, in a bid to decrease the burden on scheduling staff and teaching faculty. Many manufacturers of cosmetic products, such as fillers and neuromodulators, support foundations that make products available free of charge for residency training. Such products can be used in resident injection sessions so as to decrease the cost burden to the department. Cosmetic dermatology training after office hours or on weekends may be made available for interested residents, with such times also convenient for patients.

When in-house cosmetic faculty are not available to staff resident cosmetic surgery clinics or other resident cosmetic teaching, private-practice dermatologists or volunteer faculty in the vicinity of the residency program may supervise residents, although this can be fraught because of malpractice insurance requirements. Visiting professors from other institutions can provide didactic teaching. Residents may also be encouraged to attend national professional society meetings (eg, ASDS) that offer in-depth coursework in cosmetic procedures; additionally both American Academy of Dermatology and ASDS offer annual cosmetic dermatology courses particularly geared to residents. Registration and travel expenses associated with these courses and professional meetings are frequently free for residents, with the cost covered by the professional societies through donations received. Several professional societies also offer didactic materials, such as books (eg, ASDS primers on cosmetic and dermatologic surgery) and free on-line lectures on cosmetic topics for residents. Preceptorships available through professional societies (eg, American Society for Laser Medicine and Surgery, ASDS, and Women's Dermatologic Society) cover the expenses for residents to travel to observe cosmetic dermatologists at other centers for a week or longer.

One well-established means for overcoming gaps pertaining to knowledge and skill is completion of additional postresidency training.[6] Such training may take the form of an ASDS-approved fellowship in cosmetic dermatologic surgery. Inaugurated in 2013, this 1-year fellowship includes the range of cosmetic procedures performed by dermatologists, and ensures that every fellow independently completes at least several hundred cases across different cosmetic procedure categories.

REFERENCES

1. Ibrahimi OA, Bangash H, Green L, et al. Perceptions of expertise in cutaneous surgery and cosmetic procedures: what primary care physicians think. Dermatol Surg 2012;38(10):1645–51.

2. Alam M, Ibrahim O, Nodzenski M, et al. Adverse events associated with Mohs micrographic surgery: multicenter prospective cohort study of 20,821 cases at 23 centers. JAMA Dermatol 2013;149(12):1378–85.

3. Resneck JS Jr, Kimball AB. Who else is providing care in dermatology practices? Trends in the use of nonphysician clinicians. J Am Acad Dermatol 2008; 58(2):211–6.

4. Choudhry S, Kim NA, Gillum J, et al. State medical board regulation of minimally invasive cosmetic procedures. J Am Acad Dermatol 2012;66(1):86–91.

5. Jalian HR, Jalian CA, Avram MM. Increased risk of litigation associated with laser surgery by nonphysician operators. JAMA Dermatol 2014;150(4):407–11.

6. Jalian HR, Jalian CA, Avram MM. Common causes of injury and legal action in laser surgery. JAMA Dermatol 2013;149(2):188–93.

7. Bangash HK, Ibrahimi OA, Green LJ, et al. Who do you prefer? A study of public preferences for health care provider type in performing cutaneous surgery and cosmetic procedures in the United States. Dermatol Surg 2014;40(6):671–8.

8. Lee EH, Nehal KS, Dusza SW, et al. Procedural dermatology training during dermatology residency: a survey of third-year dermatology residents. J Am Acad Dermatol 2011;64(3):475–83, 483.e1–5.

9. Reichel JL, Peirson RP, Berg D. Teaching and evaluation of surgical skills in dermatology: results of a survey. Arch Dermatol 2004;140(11):1365–9.

Practice and Educational Gaps in Light, Laser, and Energy Treatments

Murad Alam, MD, MSCI, MBA[a,b,c,]*, Abigail Waldman, MD[a],
Keyvan Nouri, MD[d], M. Laurin Council, MD[e], Todd V. Cartee, MD[f]

KEYWORDS

- Laser dermatology • Cosmetic dermatology • Practice gaps

KEY POINTS

- This article discusses current practice in laser dermatology, the gaps in practice, and recommendations for improvement.
- As is the case with other areas of cosmetic dermatology, there is a rapid development of new laser and light devices with limited epidemiologic data available to inform best practice.
- The high fixed cost associated with new laser devices, limited space available in some practices, and inconsistent training may limit the adoption of needed therapies. Improving research in this area; training opportunities for physicians, residents, and staff; and cost-effective laser/light device rentals programs could improve quality of current practice.

The first use of lasers in medicine was for the treatment of dermatologic disease by Leon Goldman in 1961.[1] Goldman went on to become the director of dermatology at the University of Cincinnati, and the first president of the American Society for Laser Medicine and Surgery. Further research advances in laser dermatology and surgery were spearheaded by R. Rox Anderson at the Wellman Institute for Photomedicine at Harvard University, and his clinical counterpart, Kenneth A. Arndt, who also wrote the first textbooks in the field. Dermatology continues to be a major repository of laser expertise within medicine. In recent years, the dermatology laser field has enlarged to include broadband light as well as other energy sources, such as radiofrequency and therapeutic ultrasound. Clinical dermatology applications of lasers and energy devices have grown, and more dermatologists than ever before own and use instruments.

PART I. PRACTICE GAPS (IN CLINICAL DERMATOLOGY PRACTICE)
Best Practice

Best practices for laser, light, and energy device procedures are largely similar to best practices for cosmetic dermatologic surgery (see previous section) (Box 1). Additional best practices relevant

Financial Disclosures and Conflicts of Interest: None.
Funding Support: This publication was supported by Merz Center for Quality and Outcomes Research in Dermatologic Surgery and the IMPROVED (Measurement of Priority Outcome Variables in Dermatologic Surgery) group.
[a] Micrographic Surgery and Dermatology Oncology, Department of Dermatology, Feinberg School of Medicine, Northwestern University, 676 North St. Clair Street, Suite 1600, Chicago, IL 60611, USA; [b] Department of Otolaryngology, Feinberg School of Medicine, Northwestern University, 676 North St. Clair Street, Suite 1600, Chicago, IL 60611, USA; [c] Department of Surgery, Feinberg School of Medicine, Northwestern University, 676 North St. Clair Street, Suite 1600, Chicago, IL 60611, USA; [d] Department of Dermatology and Cutaneous Surgery, University of Miami Miller School of Medicine, 1475 NW 12th Avenue, Miami, FL 33136, USA; [e] Division of Dermatology, Department of Internal Medicine, Washington University in St Louis, 969 Mason Rd., Suite 200, St Louis, MO 63141, USA; [f] Department of Dermatology, Pennsylvania State University, Penn State Milton S. Hershey Medical Center, 500 University Drive, UPC 1, Suite 100, Hershey, PA 17033, USA
* Corresponding author. Department of Dermatology, 676 North St. Clair Street, Suite 1600, Chicago, IL 60611.
E-mail address: m-alam@northwestern.edu

Dermatol Clin 34 (2016) 347–352
http://dx.doi.org/10.1016/j.det.2016.03.002
0733-8635/16/$ – see front matter © 2016 Elsevier Inc. All rights reserved.

Box 1
Laser, light, and energy treatments: practice gaps

Best Practice

- Availability of appropriate protective eyewear for patients and operators, and other in-room safety protocols.
- Scheduled preventive maintenance of devices.
- Designation of a laser safety officer and training of all personnel who work with lasers and energy devices.
- Identifying contraindications for laser therapy and lower energy treatments to reduce risk when appropriate.

How Current Practices Differ from Best Practice

- Slow or variable adoption of novel device technologies with potential inability to offer a range of device options for different patients.
- Variability in staff training in laser safety, maintenance procedures, and operating procedures.
- Relative dearth of epidemiologic information regarding the procedures sought by patients, their ability to access these procedures, and their satisfaction after treatment.

Barriers to Best Practice Implementation

- Substantial fixed cost of acquiring lasers and energy devices, and the associated difficulty in covering these hardware costs in low-volume laser practices.
- Limited space in-office for storage of bulky lasers, with this being a particular issue in urban centers.
- Shortage of time available to research new devices, acquire new laser training and skills, incorporate new devices and procedures into the practice, and retrain all relevant staff.
- Reluctance to decrease general dermatology practice time to accommodate laser procedures.
- Inaccessibility or unavailability of reliable authorities or consultants who can advise dermatologists on upgrading their hardware and retraining themselves and their staff in a pragmatic, cost-efficient manner.
- Educational and training options for cutaneous laser and device surgery are not well advertised. There is no central repository that lists or vets all laser courses, programs of relevant professional societies, online educational modules, and preceptorship and fellowship opportunities.
- Limited research funding and inherent difficulties in comparing laser procedures side by side.

Strategies to Overcome Barriers

- Making laser use more cost-effective for dermatologists who have lower volume practices via rental or leasing programs that offer the latest products, come with appropriate training, and allow every dermatologist who wants to provide particular procedures to be able to do so.
- Investment in research to uncover and perfect novel medical indications for laser and energy devices.
- Easily accessible, comprehensive list of training opportunities.
- A match process for fellowships in laser and cosmetic surgery would also help advertise the availability of such more in-depth training options.

---

to lasers and light devices include (1) availability of appropriate protective eyewear for patients and operators, and other in-room safety protocols; (2) scheduled preventive maintenance of devices, often within the context of ongoing service contracts; and (3) designation of a laser safety officer and training of all personnel who work with lasers and energy devices.

Since the advent of selective laser devices in 1983, lasers and energy devices have become increasingly specialized, with certain wavelengths, pulse durations, and underlying technologies used for specific dermatologic indications. Best practice among full-service laser practices is to have available on-site a suite of devices that collectively are able to address all patient complaints amenable to energy treatment. This does not mean laser practices are expected to own every dermatologic energy device. Rather, the leading practices have one or more devices of each technological type, and for each indication.

Laser treatments pose significant risks to patients: pigmentary abnormality, scar, and ocular injury.[2-5] Darker skinned patients or tanned light-skinned patients may not be good candidates for certain laser treatments, and best practice entails identifying these contraindications and precluding inappropriate treatments. Some devices, and lower energy treatments, may reduce the risk of hyperpigmentation or hypopigmentation in susceptible patients. Scar risk is associated with high-energy treatments, resurfacing treatments that ablate or remove the epidermis and dermis, and excessive heat delivery to the skin. Using lower settings, especially in less privileged sites like the neck and decollete, avoiding pulse stacking or overlapping, and appropriate cooling (eg, spray cooling, contact cooling, air cooling) can avoid thermal injuries that can cause blistering, delayed wound healing, and scar. Best practice includes managing pigmentation and scar risk to ensure that such outcomes are uncommon to rare.

Dermatologists using lasers are well-trained, having acquired theoretic and practical expertise on the use of these devices through residency training, postresidency coursework and professional meeting attendance, and in some cases, fellowship training in cutaneous laser surgery.[6,7]

Current Practice

A number of realities cause current practice to deviate from best practice. The expense of acquisition and maintenance of modern lasers compels many practices to offer only a subset of the most highly used laser and energy device treatments. In practices in which lasers are a small part of the total practice volume, not all personnel may be trained in laser use and safety, and dedicated laser rooms may not be available. To minimize risk of adverse events, some practices may choose to limit treatment of darker skinned patients, or to avoid resurfacing treatments that require copious postoperative wound care and can be associated with delayed healing and scar. Competence in managing severe or unusual adverse events may be limited by laser procedure volume, with lower throughput practitioners exhibiting relatively less experience and skill in this area, as these outcomes are uncommon. Virtually all dermatologists performing laser procedures are well trained, having obtained this training in residency and beyond; not all have completed fellowship training in lasers and energy devices.

Some procedures are delivered by dermatologists, and some by staff, such as midlevel nonphysician providers, trained by them and under their direct supervision. Some dermatologists are more likely to delegate procedures. Degree of allowable delegation may also be influenced by state laws.[7]

Gaps and Their Classification

Gaps include (1) slow or variable adoption of novel device technologies (gap type: skill and practice); (2) failure to offer a range of device options such that most patient-requested indications can be satisfied (gap type: attitude and practice); (3) less trained staff who may not all be expert in laser safety, maintenance procedures, and operating procedures (gap type: knowledge and skill); (4) decreased willingness to offer high-risk procedures, like resurfacing and treatment of darker skinned patients (gap type: skill and practice); and (5) diminished ability to manage adverse events among less busy laser dermatologists (gap type: knowledge and skill).

Lack of fellowship training in lasers and energy devices cannot be construed as a gap, as adequate training can be acquired by other means, like residency training and postresidency coursework. However, there is a gap in that prospective laser dermatologists may not be aware of the increasing availability of laser fellowships, which have become more formalized in recent years (gap type: knowledge).

As with cosmetic dermatologic surgery, in the dermatologic laser and device field there is a relative dearth of epidemiologic information regarding the procedures sought by patients, their ability to access these procedures, and their satisfaction after treatment.[8,9] There are few reliable standardized measurement tools to assess clinical outcomes after laser procedures. Comparative effectiveness research that side by side assesses the effectiveness, cost, longevity of effect, patient acceptance, or safety of procedures for similar indications is in its infancy. These research gaps impact the knowledge available to practicing dermatologists.

Barriers and How They May Be Overcome

Barriers include (1) the substantial fixed cost of acquiring lasers and energy devices, and the associated difficulty in covering these hardware costs in low-volume laser practices; (2) limited space in-office for storage of bulky lasers, with this being a particular issue in urban centers; (3) shortage of time available to research new devices, acquire new laser training and skills, incorporate new devices and procedures into the practice, and retrain all relevant staff; (4) absence of comparative effectiveness research to support informed decisions about the relative merits of existing lasers or the utility of new technologies; (4) reluctance to decrease general dermatology practice time to accommodate laser procedures; and (5) inaccessibility or unavailability of reliable authorities or consultants who can advise dermatologists on upgrading their hardware and retraining themselves and their staff in a pragmatic, cost-efficient manner.

Laser device use is less standardized than use of other cosmetic dermatologic devices. To some extent, this lack of standardization is desirable, because settings can be tuned to the specific needs of particular patients. But for dermatologists who are less expert in laser and energy device procedures this high degree of variability can be perceived as uncertainty and risk.

Educational and training options for cutaneous laser and device surgery are not well advertised. There is no central repository that lists or vets all laser courses, programs of relevant professional societies, online educational modules, and preceptorship and fellowship opportunities. There is no fellowship match site.

From a research standpoint, barriers are similar to those applicable to cosmetic dermatologic surgery (see Waldman A, Sobanko JF, Alam M: Practice and Educational Gaps in Cosmetic Dermatologic Surgery, in this issue), with limited research funding and inherent difficulties in comparing laser procedures side by side. The technical difficulties of comparative effectiveness research in laser technology are even greater than those in general cosmetic dermatologic surgery due to the large number of adjustable laser device parameters. Varying settings like spot size, fluence, pulse duration, and cooling can result in an almost infinite number of potential combinations. Outcomes of comparisons of different energy devices therefore often hinge on the specific parameters selected rather than the intrinsic effectiveness of each device.

Overcoming these barriers will require making laser use more cost-effective for dermatologists who have lower-volume practices. Lasers and energy devices entail a large capital expense and recurring maintenance cost that may not be feasible for small cosmetic practices. Manufacturers may consider blue ribbon rental or leasing programs that offer the latest products, come with appropriate training, and allow every dermatologist who wants to provide particular procedures to be able to do so. Professional societies may also be able to support such rental programs. As with cosmetic devices and drugs, laser manufacturers may also want to invest in research to uncover and perfect novel medical indications for laser and energy devices. Expanding such indications may not only increase the pool of patients who want laser but also increase the interest of medical dermatologists in acquiring laser devices.

Group training sessions, common in cosmetic dermatology at national and regional meetings, are rare with lasers, given the numerous unique safety considerations associated with laser light. Major professional societies should investigate sponsoring laser training seminars of sufficiently small scope and hosted in venues in which live laser demonstrations would be feasible. Major professional societies or other authorities may also choose to provide a Web page that allows prospective laser dermatologists to find appropriate training opportunities. Such a listing should be comprehensive and have a detailed search function that allows users to specify exactly what type of training they are seeking in terms of time commitment, venue, subject, and level of complexity (eg, introductory, intermediate, advanced). A match process for fellowships in laser and cosmetic surgery would also help advertise the availability of such more in-depth training options.

Methods for overcoming the research barriers associated with laser and energy devices are similar to those useful in the context of cosmetic dermatologic surgery, and have been already discussed (see Waldman A, Sobanko JF, Alam M: Practice and Educational Gaps in Cosmetic Dermatologic Surgery, in this issue). Regarding the peculiar problems of laser research, namely the profusion of device parameters that must be adjusted, additional remedies are needed. Dose finding to determine optimal settings of a particular device for a specific indication is not always easy even when the investigator is unbiased and free of conflicts of interest. The Food and Drug Administration may require, or manufacturers may volunteer, additional postmarketing research to identify optimal parameters for a range of specific indications. This will help users adapt treatment technique to particular circumstances rather than to use cookie-cutter settings that may be less beneficial for some patients.

PART II. EDUCATIONAL GAPS (IN DERMATOLOGY RESIDENCY EDUCATION)
Best Practice

Best practice is that graduating residents be proficient in the performance of a range of laser and energy device procedures (**Box 2**). Technologies with which they should be familiar include broadband light, pulsed-dye laser, KTP laser, Q-switched

Box 2
Laser, light, and energy treatments: educational gaps

Best Practice

- Graduating residents should be competent to proficient in the performance of a range of laser and energy device procedures.

How Current Practices Differ from Best Practice

- Exposure and training in lasers is highly variable among residency programs. Some dermatology trainees may not be competent in the use of the entire range of cutaneous lasers and energy devices by the end of residency. These are gaps in knowledge and skill.

Barriers to Best Practice Implementation

- Time restraints and limited faculty involved in resident education on lasers.

Strategies to Overcome Barriers

- Dermatology departments should be encouraged to purchase at least a basic complement of laser and energy devices. This can be justified to hospital capital allocation committees as necessary for residency education and likely to be revenue generating, or at least revenue neutral.

- The Accreditation Council for Graduate Medical Education Residency Review Committee for dermatology may also choose to increase the minimum threshold for laser proficiency in laser to include additional devices.

lasers, picoseconds lasers, alexandrite lasers, diode lasers, Nd:YAG lasers, fractional resurfacing lasers, fully ablative lasers, endovenous lasers and radiofrequency, externally applied ultrasound, externally applied radiofrequency, insertional needle radiofrequency, and cryolipolysis. Indications they should understand include treatment of vascular lesions, pigmented lesions, tattoos, hirsutism, fine lines and wrinkles, loose skin, leg veins, and excess fat.

Current Practice

Current practice is highly variable. As with cosmetic dermatologic surgery, some residency programs ensure resident competence in many to most categories of cutaneous laser devices for many to most indications. Usually, these programs are based in dermatology departments with a large laser practice staffed by one or more dedicated laser dermatologists. In some other programs, laser education in residency consists of some hands-on training on a small number of devices for a limited range of indications. Some programs may also provide lectures and didactic information on other laser devices and indications.

Gaps and Their Classification

Some dermatology trainees may not be competent in the use of the entire range of cutaneous lasers and energy devices by the end of residency. These are gaps in knowledge and skill.

Barriers and How They May Be Overcome

Barriers include limited time to train residents in laser procedures, as well as a dearth of full-time laser dermatology faculty in dermatology departments supporting residency programs. As of this writing, the Accreditation Council for Graduate Medical Education (ACGME) dermatology residency requirements require laser proficiency only in the use of pulsed-dye laser. Observation of certain procedures or didactic training on particular advanced procedures is accepted in lieu of hands-on proficiency. Finally, leadership in some dermatology departments and residency programs continue to harbor a bias against training in laser dermatology, which may be viewed as secondary in importance to medical dermatology.

Means for overcoming these barriers are similar to those for addressing barriers to training for cosmetic dermatologic surgery (see Waldman A, Sobanko JF, Alam M: Practice and Educational Gaps in Cosmetic Dermatologic Surgery, in this issue). In addition, because it is difficult to impart proficiency in laser use without devices being available in-house, dermatology departments should be encouraged to purchase at least a basic complement of laser and energy devices and/or supplement with a rental agreement to provide access to a wider range of devices. This can be justified to hospital capital allocation committees as necessary for residency education and likely to be revenue generating, or at least revenue neutral. In most cases, interested faculty will need to develop a formal business plan to have a reasonable likelihood of obtaining the necessary capital funding. The ACGME Residency Review Committee for dermatology may also choose to increase the minimum threshold for laser proficiency to include 2 or 3 additional devices, such as broadband light, pigment lasers, and resurfacing devices.

REFERENCES

1. Goldman L. Future of laser dermatology. Lasers Surg Med 1998;22(1):3–8.

2. Lolis M, Dunbar SW, Goldberg DJ, et al. Patient safety in procedural dermatology: part II. Safety related to cosmetic procedures. J Am Acad Dermatol 2015; 73(1):15–24.

3. Dudelzak J, Goldberg DJ. Laser safety. Curr Probl Dermatol 2011;42:35–9.

4. Alam M, Chaudhry NA, Goldberg LH. Vitreous floaters following use of dermatologic lasers. Dermatol Surg 2002;28(11):1088–91.

5. Alam M, Warycha M. Complications of lasers and light treatments. Dermatol Ther 2011;24(6):571–80.

6. Alam M, Dover JS, Arndt KA. Use of cutaneous lasers and light sources: appropriate training and delegation. Skin Therapy Lett 2007;12(5):5–9.

7. Alam M. Who is qualified to perform laser surgery and in what setting? Semin Plast Surg 2007;21(3): 193–200.

8. Chiang YZ, Al-Niaimi F, Madan V. Comparative efficacy and patient preference of topical anaesthetics in dermatological laser treatments and skin microneedling. J Cutan Aesthet Surg 2015;8(3):143–6.

9. Bangash HK, Ibrahimi OA, Green LJ, et al. Who do you prefer? A study of public preferences for health care provider type in performing cutaneous surgery and cosmetic procedures in the United States. Dermatol Surg 2014;40(6):671–8.

Practice Gaps in Dermatology
Melanocytic Lesions and Melanoma

Maria L. Marino, MD[a], Cristina Carrera, MD, PhD[a,b], Michael A. Marchetti, MD[a,*,1], Ashfaq A. Marghoob, MD[a,*,1]

KEYWORDS

- Dermoscopy • Digital dermoscopy • Sequential digital dermoscopy imaging
- Early melanoma diagnosis • Melanoma • Nevi • Reflectance confocal microscopy
- Total body photography

KEY POINTS

- Good practices for melanoma diagnosis include strategies to detect new or changing skin lesions.
- Dermoscopy, total body photography, sequential digital dermoscopy imaging, and reflectance confocal microscopy are at present most relevant to identifying and evaluating new or changing skin lesions.
- The use of these noninvasive imaging technologies is particularly useful when screening individuals with high melanocytic nevus counts and atypical/complex nevus phenotypes for melanoma.
- Barriers such as lack of training and confidence, personal beliefs, and economical and logistical constraints have prevented the widespread use of those tools.
- Patient-driven health care aided by technology and complemented by teledermatology will likely rapidly alter the landscape of melanoma screening within the next decade.

IMPORTANCE OF NEW OR CHANGING MELANOCYTIC LESIONS

Despite increased public awareness of skin cancer and of the harmful effects of ultraviolet radiation (UVR), cutaneous melanoma incidence and mortality continue to increase in the United States. In 2015, approximately 73,870 people will be diagnosed with and 9940 will die of invasive melanoma.[1] Although there have been recent improvements in the treatment of metastatic melanoma,[2] early detection remains the most important strategy to reduce mortality. Evidence supporting this approach includes the recent population-based screening efforts in Germany, with initial results in the state of Schleswig-Holstein suggesting a nearly 50% decrease in melanoma mortality associated with skin cancer screening through total body skin examinations (TBSEs).[3]

Many factors are recognized as important to the diagnosis of melanoma,[4] including the identification of new or changing lesions. In 2004, the letter "E" was appended to the ABCD (Asymmetry, irregular Borders, more than one or uneven distribution of Color, or a large [greater than 6 mm] Diameter) mnemonic to highlight the importance of change in a melanocytic lesion as an important diagnostic criterion of melanoma.[5,6] Similarly, the Glasgow 7-point checklist

Financial Disclosures: None reported.
[a] Dermatology Service, Department of Medicine, Memorial Sloan Kettering Cancer Center, 16 East 60th Street, New York, NY 10022, USA; [b] Melanoma Unit, Department of Dermatology, Hospital Clinic, IDIBAPS, CIBERER, University of Barcelona, Villarroel 170, Barcelona 08036, Spain
[1] Contributed equally.
* Corresponding authors.
E-mail addresses: marchetm@mskcc.org; marghooa@mskcc.org

Dermatol Clin 34 (2016) 353–362
http://dx.doi.org/10.1016/j.det.2016.03.003
0733-8635/16/$ – see front matter © 2016 Elsevier Inc. All rights reserved.

derm.theclinics.com

places significant importance on changes in size, shape, and color of skin lesions as major signs of melanoma.[7] The fact that most melanomas (~65%) arise de novo and are not contiguously associated with a melanocytic nevus underscores the importance of identifying new lesions in addition to changing lesions during TBSEs to maximize diagnostic sensitivity for melanoma. As the associated potential harms of skin cancer screening, in particular overdiagnosis, are increasingly recognized,[8,9] identification of truly dynamic lesions with real potential for progression to metastatic and fatal disease may have the greatest short-term potential to limit harvesting of indolent and/or nonprogressive cancers.

Emphasis on detection and subsequent biopsy of changing skin lesions, however, may lead to a decrease in diagnostic accuracy for melanoma. A surrogate marker of positive predictive value is number needed to excise (NNE), which is the number of benign melanocytic lesions removed for every confirmed melanoma. Estimates in Europe and the United States of the NNE in children and adolescents are reported to range from 594 to 696, which are attributed to relying on change alone as an indication for biopsy.[10–13] Nevogenesis is recognized as a highly dynamic process during life, with significant nevus volatility in younger individuals (ie, nevus growth, appearance, and disappearance).[14–16] Even in adults, change alone in a skin lesion is not specific for the diagnosis of melanoma, and the appearance of new nevi is relatively common.[13,17] Conditions such as body growth, weight gain, pregnancy, or UVR exposure can also lead to recognized benign changes in melanocytic lesions.[18,19]

CURRENT BEST PRACTICE

Good practices for melanoma diagnosis therefore include, but are not limited to, strategies to detect new and/or changing lesions and to determine if these findings warrant skin biopsy. The use of noninvasive imaging technologies, such as dermoscopy, total body photography (TBP), sequential digital dermoscopy imaging (SDDI), and reflectance confocal microscopy (RCM), are at present most relevant to identifying and evaluating new and changing skin lesions during screening examinations, particularly in individuals with high melanocytic nevus counts and atypical/complex nevus phenotypes.[20]

Use of TBP images by physicians and patients during TBSEs and skin self-examinations (SSEs), respectively, allow for identification of new lesions and macroscopic changes in existing skin lesions (Fig. 1). Physicians who routinely use TBP during skin examinations argue that its use improves sensitivity and specificity for melanoma detection.[21–24] Use of TBP images during SSEs has been shown to improve patients' confidence in performing SSEs[25–27] and to increase patients' sensitivity for detection of new or changing skin lesions compared with performance of SSE alone without access to TBP images.[26]

After recognition of a new or changing skin lesion with TBP, dermoscopic evaluation is the next most appropriate step in evaluation. Meta-analyses have demonstrated that the use of dermoscopy by trained evaluators improves diagnostic accuracy for melanoma detection.[28–30] Access to dermoscopy reduces unnecessary biopsies of skin lesions[31,32] because most pigmented lesions will conform to a recognized benign nevus pattern.[33] The predominant nevus pattern depends on age, skin type, and the interaction between genes and the environment, such as UVR exposure. In the context of patients with many nevi, use of the dermoscopic comparative examination and the ugly duckling concept will prevent unnecessary biopsies of nevi.[19,31,32,34] Lesions with features concerning for melanoma should undergo biopsy, whereas those with equivocal but not diagnostic features could undergo SDDI and/or interrogation with RCM.

SDDI involves capturing dermoscopic images of lesions over time in order to identify changes concerning for melanoma and can be used in 2 complementary ways. The first method involves repeating dermoscopic images of skin lesions at regular intervals for detailed comparative analysis, which when combined with TBP has been referred to as "digital follow-up"[35,36] and has been shown to enable recognition of melanomas that lack diagnostic clinical or dermoscopic features at baseline evaluation (Fig. 2).[37,38] SDDI can also be used as a second-level screening evaluation of specific lesions with borderline features. When used in this manner, SDDI dramatically reduces the number of biopsies of benign lesions compared with use of dermoscopy alone (Fig. 3).[39] Access to SDDI compared with dermoscopy alone has also been associated with a 35% reduction in the cost per melanoma excised in a 1-year retrospective observational study in Belgium.[40]

A 5-year prospective observation study of 311 patients in Australia at "extreme high risk" for melanoma demonstrates the complementary effectiveness of TBP, dermoscopy, and SDDI in the diagnosis of melanoma.[41] After a median follow-up of 3.5 years, 70 of 75 primary melanomas detected in this cohort were either in situ

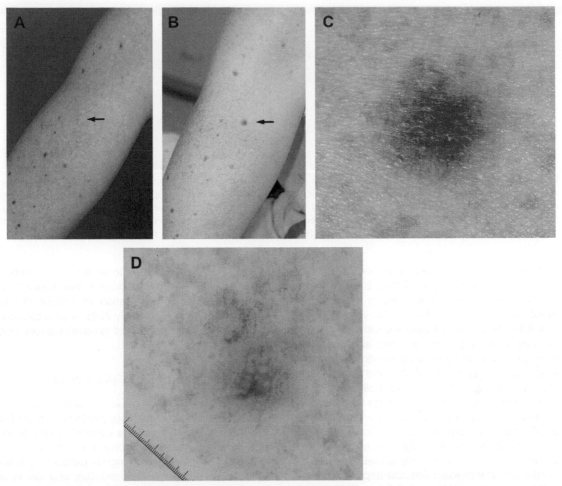

Fig. 1. Total body photography aids identification of changing skin lesions. A lesion on the arm was noted to increase in size (*B, arrow*) during follow-up skin examination when compared with a baseline photograph of the lesion captured 4 years before (*A, arrow*). Close-up clinical (*C*) and nonpolarized dermoscopy (*D*) images reveal a featureless tan-pink homogenous papule surrounded by solar lentigines. Skin biopsy showed invasive melanoma with maximum thickness of 0.3 mm arising in association with a nevus.

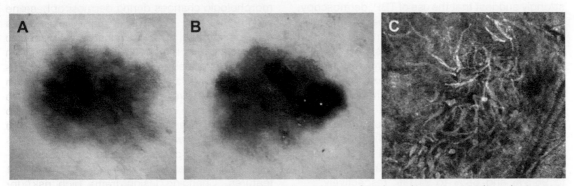

Fig. 2. Sequential digital dermoscopic imaging allows recognition of early melanomas. Baseline dermoscopy image (*A*) shows peripheral reticular pattern with central hyperpigmentation, consistent with banal nevus. After 6 months, focal hyperpigmentation (*asterisk*) was noted on repeat dermoscopic imaging (*B*). Reflectance confocal microscopic examination of the area of focal hyperpigmentation (*C*) showed infiltration of pagetoid dendritic and roundish cells in the epidermis, which was confirmed by histopathology of skin biopsy to be melanoma in situ arising in association with a nevus.

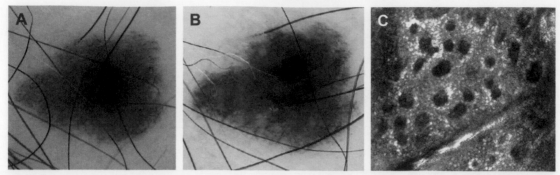

Fig. 3. Reflectance confocal microscopy can help prevent unnecessary skin biopsies. Sequential digital dermoscopy imaging of a skin lesion revealed symmetric enlargement as well as the appearance of dots, focal hyperpigmentation, and disruption of the network (B) when compared with baseline (A), suggestive of malignancy. (C) Reflectance confocal microscopy showed edged papillae and ringed pattern with hyperefractile cells, typical of lentiginous melanocytic nevi. Skin biopsy confirmed lentiginous melanocytic nevus.

or 1-mm or thinner invasive melanomas. Furthermore, 39.3% and 37.7% of after-baseline melanomas were detected exclusively or aided by SDDI and TBP, respectively. The very low NNE of 4.4:1 reflects that surveillance with this protocol did not lead to excess biopsies and compares favorably to recently published estimates of NNE in skin cancer specialist (8.7:1) and nonspecialist (29.4:1) clinics.[10] Salerni and colleagues[36] reported similar overall effectiveness in melanoma screening using TBP, dermoscopy, and SDDI in a 10-year retrospective observational study of 618 patients in Spain at high risk for melanoma. In this study, 53.3% (n = 53) of melanomas were in situ, and the median Breslow depth of invasive melanomas (n = 45) was 0.5 mm.[36] Although neither study was designed to investigate if intensive screening for melanoma with these imaging techniques is associated with reduced mortality or melanoma overdiagnosis, these studies as well as a recent meta-analysis on the topic[28] strongly suggest that the use of TBP, dermoscopy, and SDDI to identify and evaluate new or changing skin lesions permits early melanoma diagnosis at curable stages with low NNE ratios.

New or changing skin lesions with equivocal features after dermoscopic or SDDI examination can undergo analysis with RCM, which noninvasively allows for cellular assessment of the epidermis and superficial dermis at a resolution approaching histologic detail (see Fig. 2; Fig. 4). The reported sensitivity and specificity of RCM for melanoma among experts are estimated to range from 91% to 96.5% and 68% to 94.1%, respectively.[42,43] Used as a second-level screening test, RCM has been shown to improve diagnostic accuracy for melanoma and to prevent unnecessary biopsies of benign lesions.[18,42,44,45] RCM may be particularly useful for evaluation of amelanotic, facial, or

dermoscopically nonspecific lesions.[42,44] Studies have specifically demonstrated the impact of RCM as a screening evaluation after SDDI. In this setting, it can prevent nearly 70% of unnecessary biopsies of benign nevi found to have changes that warrant removal.[45,46]

Relevant Dermoscopic Changes During Follow-up

Detected changes in melanocytic lesions must be interpreted depending on a patient's phenotype, risk markers, and predominant dermoscopic pattern. The interval of change is particularly relevant; any short-term (0–3 months) change in a lesion on an adult should be of concern and biopsy strongly considered. Exceptions could include physiologic changes during pregnancy or pubertal growth, recent intense UVR exposure, or laser depilation.

Nevi and melanomas can display similar morphologic changes during dermoscopic monitoring and may even grow at similar rates.[47] Indeed, studies have demonstrated that nevi and melanomas removed during SDDI are often clinically and dermoscopically indistinguishable and that change alone permitted melanoma identification. However, the most relevant changes associated with melanoma during SDDI are asymmetric enlargement, appearance of focal or eccentric new structures (ie, "dermoscopic island"), or the appearance of atypical focal dermoscopic features such as vessels or regression features. Changing lesions with features concerning for melanoma should undergo biopsy, whereas lesions with equivocal features can undergo RCM or repeated dermoscopic imaging over a longer or sometimes indefinite time interval (Fig. 5).

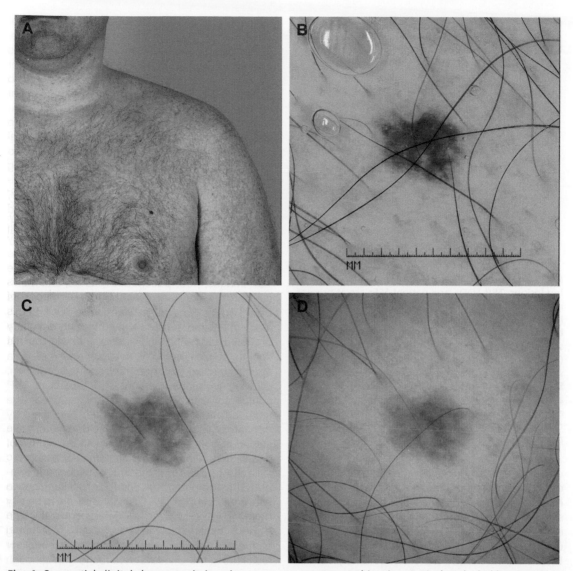

Fig. 4. Sequential digital dermoscopic imaging prevents unnecessary biopsies. An isolated, darkly pigmented macule (eg, "ugly duckling") was found on the chest of a 44-year-old man with a history of 2 invasive melanomas (*A*). Baseline nonpolarized dermoscopy (*B*) shows a reticular network without any melanoma-specific criteria. Repeat nonpolarized imaging at 3 months (*C*) and 6 months (*D*) revealed gradual lightening in pigmentation but no relevant changes concerning for melanoma.

CURRENT PRACTICE

Use of TBP to monitor patients with atypical/ dysplastic nevi began in the late 1980s.[48] By 1992, 41% of US residency programs reported use of TBP.[49] In 2000, 62% of dermatologists in academic institutions stated that they use TBP, and in 2010, this value increased to 71%.[50] Rice and colleagues[51] surveyed 49 US dermatology departments in 2010 and found that 33 (67%) used TBP as a screening method; of those who used TBP, 11 (33%) used digital TBP alone, 11 (33%) used digital with printed images of TBP,

and 11 (33%) used printed TBP images alone. In the authors' opinion, TBP is not consistently used to evaluate patients at high risk for melanoma outside of academic centers.

Use of dermoscopy by dermatologists worldwide has increased considerably since introduction in the 1980s. Although formal statistics are not readily available, it is commonly accepted that the over-whelming majority of dermatologists in Europe and Australia use dermoscopy and SDDI on a routine basis. Approximately 95% of French[52] and 98% of Australian[53,54] dermatologists recently reported

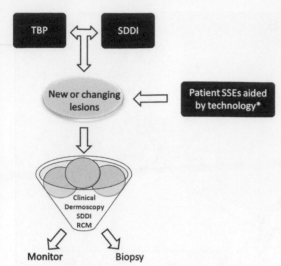

Fig. 5. Identification and evaluation of new or changing lesions. TBP, SDDI, and patient SSEs are at present most suited to detection of new or changing lesions. In the future, patients may perform SSEs aided by mobile-phone technology that includes dermoscopy, SDDI, and automated image analysis software (*asterisk*). Once detected, new or changing lesions should undergo clinical and dermoscopic examination. SDDI and RCM can be applied in equivocal lesions, if available. Ultimately, the decision to monitor or biopsy a skin lesion is made after assessing all available information, including patient concern, patient history, and physician experience/comfort.

using dermoscopy in nationwide surveys. Uptake of dermoscopy in other countries, such as the United Kingdom and United States, has been appreciably slower. A study in the United Kingdom showed an increase from 54% of dermatologists reporting regular use in 2003% to 86% in 2012.[55] Surveys in the United States showed a prevalence of any dermoscopy use by dermatologists to be 23%, 17.4%, and 48% in the years 2002, 2005, and 2009, respectively, suggesting an increase in adoption.[56–58] More recently in 2013, 80.7% of American dermatologists reported use of dermoscopy, but only 31.3% reported performing dermoscopy on all pigmented lesions and 49.3% reported using SDDI.[59]

No data exist to the authors' knowledge that estimates current practice patterns regarding (a) the combined use of dermoscopy, SDDI, and TBP; and (b) RCM, but they estimate that these techniques are limited to select academic centers with established pigmented lesion clinics.

PRACTICE AND EDUCATIONAL BARRIERS AND FACILITATORS

Multiple factors have prevented more widespread adoption of TBP to monitor patients at high risk for melanoma. Some dermatologists argue TBP is not a helpful tool beyond clinical examination alone, given the absence of randomized clinical trials evaluating the use of TBP. Physicians cite other barriers including the additional time required to perform a TBSE with TBP, lack of reimbursement for the examination, and logistical/financial constraints, such as the need to obtain software to securely organize and store patients' digital images. US dermatology residents have reported little emphasis on learning how to use TBP during training, and as many as 67.4% would prefer additional education.[50] From the patient perspective, TBP is often not covered by insurance plans and may lead to significant out-of-pocket expenses. In some geographic locations, there is simply poor access to imaging centers that provide TBP. In addition, the time required to capture TBP images, poor patient acceptance, and medical liability have been described as barriers to its use.[50] To facilitate more widespread use of TBP, medical insurance plans should include coverage of TBP imaging for individuals with high nevus counts, atypical/complex nevus phenotypes, or a strong personal history of melanoma. In addition, allowing for reimbursement of TBSE using TBP compared with TBSE alone may address the time, logistical, and financial constraints cited by dermatologists. Dermatology residency curricula should also include specific training on the use of and evidence for TBP in melanoma screening.

Lack of proper training and confidence are reported as common reasons for physicians not to use dermoscopy.[50,55] Training with an expert in dermoscopy has been shown to correlate with higher confidence levels when evaluating pigmented lesions.[60] A survey of chief dermatology residents in the United States found that although 94% reported using dermoscopy, only 48% had been trained by a specialist.[60] From 2000 to 2010, US dermatology residency programs reported a decrease in the number of dermoscopy experts in their programs.[50] The lack of mentorship in dermoscopy was associated in 2 recent surveys with dermatology residents reporting poor satisfaction with their dermoscopy training.[61,62] Despite meta-analyses and clinical practice guidelines supporting the use of dermoscopy in evaluating pigmented skin lesions, some physicians question the benefits of dermoscopy, including its ability to increase sensitivity of melanoma diagnosis in real practice[63] and its effect on patient outcomes, specifically overall mortality. These concerns appear to have decreased in recent years; in a survey in 2000, 41% of responders found dermoscopy not a helpful tool. In contrast, a survey in 2009 showed that number to be 23.1%.[50] For some practitioners, dermoscopy use can initially increase anxiety levels,[50] but it has been shown that after an 18-month learning curve, a general dermatologist can achieve a similar NNE as a pigmented lesion specialist.[64] The additional time required to perform a TBSE with dermoscopy has also been cited as a reason not to use dermoscopy. In one study, the median time needed for TBSE without dermoscopy was half as long as with dermoscopy and was in direct proportion to the patient's total lesion count.[65]

To address these concerns, dermatology training programs should include specific training and competency examinations in dermoscopy and facilitate attendance of regional, national, or international dermoscopy lectures given by dermoscopy experts. National dermatology training curricula should emphasize learning dermoscopy, and national certifying examinations in dermatology should measure proficiency in dermoscopic diagnosis. In order to promote use of dermoscopy, Australia, New Zealand, Germany, and Italy, among other countries, have issued clinical guidelines strongly recommending training in and use of dermoscopy for examination of pigmented skin lesions.[66] Knowledge of the dermoscopic evaluation of skin lesions, however, is not at present formally recommended by any US authority.

Barriers to use of SDDI include lack of knowledge regarding the utility of the technique and lack of training in image analysis. Proper use of SDDI is estimated to require 10 to 20 hours of training.[67] In addition, the need for proper equipment (ie, camera, computer), imaging software, and photographers creates logistical and financial barriers for physicians. There is an urgent need for industry to produce more user-friendly software and less expensive imaging hardware to facilitate a physician's ability to use SDDI. Other barriers include lack of reimbursement for physicians who use the technique, lack of imaging standardization for comparative analysis, and lack of imaging exchangeability across physicians due to incompatible software. Finally, concerns have been raised about the potential to observe a melanoma rather than biopsy it at baseline or even miss a melanoma diagnosis if a patient fails to return for follow-up examinations. In the authors' practice (M.M. and A.M.), SDDI of specific lesions is recorded and tracked in a manner analogous to a skin biopsy, and a patient is contacted upon failure return for follow-up examination(s). Integration of data among software platforms (ie, pathology results, patient scheduling, imaging, patient portals) could facilitate care providers' ability to perform SDDI and engage patients in health care outcomes.

The primary barriers for use of RCM are equipment costs and the training and expertise required for image analysis. Specialists in RCM have estimated the necessary case training required for proficiency of evaluation of melanocytic skin lesions to be approximately 4000 cases (Giovanni Pellacani, Personal communication, 2016). Furthermore, the opportunity costs of time and personnel currently required for performing the procedure and interpreting the images in a busy practice limit the applicability of RCM as a sequential screening test to academic centers. To address these issues, the cost of the technology must continue to decrease, and there must be greater access to training materials, beginning at the resident level. In addition, technical advances such as automated detection of skin microanatomy and enhanced imaging contrast could facilitate the ability and decrease the time required of users to interpret images.

Finally, patients are increasingly assuming a more direct role in their health care and have recently been reported to self-detect melanoma using dermoscopy.[68] The rapid development of mobile-phone technology, including direct-to-consumer health applications (or "apps") and higher-quality cameras, already permits patient-initiated TBP and tracking of individual skin lesions using sequential clinical photography. With the recent introduction of low-cost ($\sim$\$80) dermatoscopes that attach to mobile phones,[69] patients are now able to economically perform SDDI and send dermoscopic images of concerning skin lesions to their health care providers. Additional research will be needed to optimize patient safety and privacy as well as the ability of laypersons to identify clinically relevant skin lesions and to capture adequate-quality images.[70–73] Patient-driven health care aided by technology and complemented by teledermatology will likely rapidly alter the landscape of melanoma screening within the next decade and improve early detection efforts.

SUMMARY

Identification of new or changing skin lesions is an important component of optimizing melanoma screening. Use of noninvasive technologies such as TBP, dermoscopy, SDDI, and RCM are currently best practice for detection of new or changing lesions. Many barriers exist that prevent more widespread adoption and use of these screening techniques, resulting in practice gaps, which may result in delayed melanoma diagnosis and unnecessary skin biopsies. Multiple factors contribute to the barriers discussed in this review, and it will require a coordinated effort from industry, government, health care organizations, dermatologists, and patients themselves to over-come these barriers and improve melanoma detection worldwide.

REFERENCES

1. Siegel RL, Miller KD, Jemal A. Cancer statistics, 2015. CA Cancer J Clin 2015;65:5–29.
2. Niezgoda A, Niezgoda P, Czajkowski R. Novel approaches to treatment of advanced melanoma: a review on targeted therapy and immunotherapy. Biomed Res Int 2015;2015:851387.
3. Katalinic A, Waldmann A, Weinstock MA, et al. Does skin cancer screening save lives?: an observational study comparing trends in melanoma mortality in regions with and without screening. Cancer 2012; 118:5395–402.
4. Marghoob AA, Scope A. The complexity of diagnosing melanoma. J Invest Dermatol 2009;129: 11–3.
5. Abbasi NR, Shaw HM, Rigel DS, et al. Early diagnosis of cutaneous melanoma: revisiting the ABCD criteria. JAMA 2004;292:2771–6.
6. Tsao H, Olazagasti JM, Cordoro KM, et al. Early detection of melanoma: reviewing the ABCDEs. J Am Acad Dermatol 2015;72:717–23.
7. MacKie RM. Clinical recognition of early invasive malignant melanoma. BMJ 1990;301:1005–6.
8. Welch HG, Woloshin S, Schwartz LM. Skin biopsy rates and incidence of melanoma: population based ecological study. BMJ 2005;331:481.
9. Swerlick RA, Chen S. The melanoma epidemic: more apparent than real? Mayo Clin Proc 1997;72: 559–64.
10. Argenziano G, Cerroni L, Zalaudek I, et al. Accuracy in melanoma detection: a 10-year multicenter survey. J Am Acad Dermatol 2012;67:54–9.
11. Oliveria SA, Selvam N, Mehregan D, et al. Biopsies of nevi in children and adolescents in the United States, 2009 through 2013. JAMA Dermatol 2015; 151:447–8.
12. Cohen B. To biopsy or not to biopsy changing moles in children and adolescents: are we removing too many pigmented nevi in this age group?: comment on "Variables predicting change in benign melanocytic nevi undergoing short-term dermoscopic imaging". Arch Dermatol 2011;147: 659–60.
13. Oliveria SA, Yagerman SE, Jaimes N, et al. Clinical and dermoscopic characteristics of new naevi in adults: results from a cohort study. Br J Dermatol 2013;169:848–53.
14. Scope A, Dusza SW, Marghoob AA, et al. Clinical and dermoscopic stability and volatility of melanocytic nevi in a population-based cohort of children in Framingham school system. J Invest Dermatol 2011;131:1615–21.
15. Moscarella E, Zalaudek I, Cerroni L, et al. Excised melanocytic lesions in children and adolescents—a 10-year survey. Br J Dermatol 2012;167:368–73.
16. Wu X, Fonseca M, Marchetti MA, et al. Longitudinally followed nevi in children and adolescents show significant size changes. Abstract #300 presented at the 2014 Society of Investigative Dermatology in Albuquerque, New Mexico. J Invest Dermatol 2014; 134(Suppl 1):S49–60.
17. Menzies SW, Stevenson ML, Altamura D, et al. Variables predicting change in benign melanocytic nevi undergoing short-term dermoscopic imaging. Arch Dermatol 2011;147:655–9.
18. Alarcon I, Carrera C, Palou J, et al. Impact of in vivo reflectance confocal microscopy on the number needed to treat melanoma in doubtful lesions. Br J Dermatol 2014;170:802–8.
19. Zalaudek I, Argenziano G, Mordente I, et al. Nevus type in dermoscopy is related to skin type in white persons. Arch Dermatol 2007;143:351–6.
20. Watts CG, Dieng M, Morton RL, et al. Clinical practice guidelines for identification, screening and follow-up of individuals at high risk of primary cutaneous melanoma: a systematic review. Br J Dermatol 2015;172:33–47.
21. Rhodes AR. Intervention strategy to prevent lethal cutaneous melanoma: use of dermatologic photography to aid surveillance of high-risk persons. J Am Acad Dermatol 1998;39:262–7.
22. Kelly JW, Yeatman JM, Regalia C, et al. A high incidence of melanoma found in patients with multiple dysplastic naevi by photographic surveillance. Med J Aust 1997;167:191–4.
23. Feit NE, Dusza SW, Marghoob AA. Melanomas detected with the aid of total cutaneous photography. Br J Dermatol 2004;150:706–14.
24. Goodson AG, Florell SR, Hyde M, et al. Comparative analysis of total body and dermatoscopic photographic monitoring of nevi in similar patient populations at risk for cutaneous melanoma. Dermatol Surg 2010;36:1087–98.
25. Yagerman S, Marghoob A. Melanoma patient self-detection: a review of efficacy of the skin self-examination and patient-directed educational efforts. Expert Rev Anticancer Ther 2013;13:1423–31.
26. Oliveria SA, Chau D, Christos PJ, et al. Diagnostic accuracy of patients in performing skin self-examination and the impact of photography. Arch Dermatol 2004;140:57–62.
27. Phelan DL, Oliveria SA, Christos PJ, et al. Skin self-examination in patients at high risk for melanoma: a pilot study. Oncol Nurs Forum 2003;30:1029–36.
28. Salerni G, Teran T, Puig S, et al. Meta-analysis of digital dermoscopy follow-up of melanocytic skin lesions: a study on behalf of the International Dermoscopy Society. J Eur Acad Dermatol Venereol 2013; 27:805–14.

29. Vestergaard ME, Macaskill P, Holt PE, et al. Dermoscopy compared with naked eye examination for the diagnosis of primary melanoma: a meta-analysis of studies performed in a clinical setting. Br J Dermatol 2008;159:669–76.

30. Bafounta ML, Beauchet A, Aegerter P, et al. Is dermoscopy (epiluminescence microscopy) useful for the diagnosis of melanoma? Results of a meta-analysis using techniques adapted to the evaluation of diagnostic tests. Arch Dermatol 2001;137:1343–50.

31. Carli P, De Giorgi V, Crocetti E, et al. Improvement of malignant/benign ratio in excised melanocytic lesions in the 'dermoscopy era': a retrospective study 1997-2001. Br J Dermatol 2004;150:687–92.

32. Carli P, de Giorgi V, Chiarugi A, et al. Addition of dermoscopy to conventional naked-eye examination in melanoma screening: a randomized study. J Am Acad Dermatol 2004;50:683–9.

33. Marghoob AA, Braun RP, Malvehy J. Atlas of dermoscopy. 2nd edition. New York: Informa Healthcare; 2012.

34. Argenziano G, Catricala C, Ardigo M, et al. Dermoscopy of patients with multiple nevi: Improved management recommendations using a comparative diagnostic approach. Arch Dermatol 2011;147:46–9.

35. Salerni G, Carrera C, Lovatto L, et al. Characterization of 1152 lesions excised over 10 years using total-body photography and digital dermatoscopy in the surveillance of patients at high risk for melanoma. J Am Acad Dermatol 2012;67:836–45.

36. Salerni G, Carrera C, Lovatto L, et al. Benefits of total body photography and digital dermatoscopy ("two-step method of digital follow-up") in the early diagnosis of melanoma in patients at high risk for melanoma. J Am Acad Dermatol 2012;67:e17–27.

37. Kittler H, Guitera P, Riedl E, et al. Identification of clinically featureless incipient melanoma using sequential dermoscopy imaging. Arch Dermatol 2006;142:1113–9.

38. Haenssle HA, Krueger U, Vente C, et al. Results from an observational trial: digital epiluminescence microscopy follow-up of atypical nevi increases the sensitivity and the chance of success of conventional dermoscopy in detecting melanoma. J Invest Dermatol 2006;126:980–5.

39. Tromme I, Sacre L, Hammouch F, et al. Availability of digital dermoscopy in daily practice dramatically reduces the number of excised melanocytic lesions: results from an observational study. Br J Dermatol 2012;167:778–86.

40. Tromme I, Devleesschauwer B, Beutels P, et al. Selective use of sequential digital dermoscopy imaging allows a cost reduction in the melanoma detection process: a Belgian study of patients with a single or a small number of atypical nevi. PLoS One 2014;9:e109339.

41. Moloney FJ, Guitera P, Coates E, et al. Detection of primary melanoma in individuals at extreme high risk: a prospective 5-year follow-up study. JAMA Dermatol 2014;150:819–27.

42. Guitera P, Pellacani G, Longo C, et al. In vivo reflectance confocal microscopy enhances secondary evaluation of melanocytic lesions. J Invest Dermatol 2009;129:131–8.

43. Longo C, Farnetani F, Ciardo S, et al. Is confocal microscopy a valuable tool in diagnosing nodular lesions? A study of 140 cases. Br J Dermatol 2013;169:58–67.

44. Pellacani G, Pepe P, Casari A, et al. Reflectance confocal microscopy as a second-level examination in skin oncology improves diagnostic accuracy and saves unnecessary excisions: a longitudinal prospective study. Br J Dermatol 2014;171:1044–51.

45. Stanganelli I, Longo C, Mazzoni L, et al. Integration of reflectance confocal microscopy in sequential dermoscopy follow-up improves melanoma detection accuracy. Br J Dermatol 2015;172:365–71.

46. Lovatto L, Carrera C, Salerni G, et al. In vivo reflectance confocal microscopy of equivocal melanocytic lesions detected by digital dermoscopy follow-up. J Eur Acad Dermatol Venereol 2015;29(10):1918–25.

47. Bajaj S, Dusza SW, Marchetti MA, et al. Growth-curve modeling of nevi with a peripheral globular pattern. JAMA Dermatol 2015;151(12):1338–45.

48. Slue W, Kopf AW, Rivers JK. Total-body photographs of dysplastic nevi. Arch Dermatol 1988;124:1239–43.

49. Shriner DL, Wagner RF Jr. Photographic utilization in dermatology clinics in the United States: a survey of university-based dermatology residency programs. J Am Acad Dermatol 1992;27:565–7.

50. Terushkin V, Oliveria SA, Marghoob AA, et al. Use of and beliefs about total body photography and dermatoscopy among US dermatology training programs: an update. J Am Acad Dermatol 2010;62:794–803.

51. Rice ZP, Weiss FJ, DeLong LK, et al. Utilization and rationale for the implementation of total body (digital) photography as an adjunct screening measure for melanoma. Melanoma Res 2010;20:417–21.

52. Moulin C, Poulalhon N, Duru G, et al. Dermoscopy use by French private practice dermatologists: a nationwide survey. Br J Dermatol 2013;168:74–9.

53. Piliouras P, Buettner P, Soyer HP. Dermoscopy use in the next generation: a survey of Australian dermatology trainees. Australas J Dermatol 2014;55:49–52.

54. Venugopal SS, Soyer HP, Menzies SW. Results of a nationwide dermoscopy survey investigating the prevalence, advantages and disadvantages of dermoscopy use among Australian dermatologists. Australas J Dermatol 2011;52:14–8.

55. Butler TD, Matin RN, Affleck AG, et al. Trends in dermoscopy use in the UK: results from surveys in 2003 and 2012. Dermatol Pract Concept 2015;5: 29–38.

56. Engasser HC, Warshaw EM. Dermatoscopy use by US dermatologists: a cross-sectional survey. J Am Acad Dermatol 2010;63:412–9, 419.e1–2.

57. Tripp JM, Kopf AW, Marghoob AA, et al. Management of dysplastic nevi: a survey of fellows of the American Academy of Dermatology. J Am Acad Dermatol 2002;46:674–82.

58. Charles CA, Yee VS, Dusza SW, et al. Variation in the diagnosis, treatment, and management of melanoma in situ: a survey of US dermatologists. Arch Dermatol 2005;141:723–9.

59. Murzaku EC, Hayan S, Rao BK. Methods and rates of dermoscopy usage: a cross-sectional survey of US dermatologists stratified by years in practice. J Am Acad Dermatol 2014;71:393–5.

60. Wu TP, Newlove T, Smith L, et al. The importance of dedicated dermoscopy training during residency: a survey of US dermatology chief residents. J Am Acad Dermatol 2013;68:1000–5.

61. Freeman SR, Greene RE, Kimball AB, et al. US dermatology residents' satisfaction with training and mentoring: survey results from the 2005 and 2006 Las Vegas Dermatology Seminars. Arch Dermatol 2008;144:896–900.

62. Freiman A, Barzilai DA, Barankin B, et al. National appraisal of dermatology residency training: a Canadian study. Arch Dermatol 2005;141:1100–4.

63. Carli P. Dermoscopy not yet shown to increase sensitivity of melanoma diagnosis in real practice. Arch Dermatol 2007;143:664–5 [author reply: 665–6].

64. Terushkin V, Warycha M, Levy M, et al. Analysis of the benign to malignant ratio of lesions biopsied by a general dermatologist before and after the adoption of dermoscopy. Arch Dermatol 2010;146: 343–4.

65. Zalaudek I, Kittler H, Marghoob AA, et al. Time required for a complete skin examination with and without dermoscopy: a prospective, randomized multicenter study. Arch Dermatol 2008;144:509–13.

66. Halpern AC, Marchetti MA, Marghoob AA. Melanoma surveillance in "high-risk" individuals. JAMA Dermatol 2014;150(8):815–6.

67. Menzies SW, Emery J, Staples M, et al. Impact of dermoscopy and short-term sequential digital dermoscopy imaging for the management of pigmented lesions in primary care: a sequential intervention trial. Br J Dermatol 2009;161:1270–7.

68. Goulart JM, Malvehy J, Puig S, et al. Dermoscopy in skin self-examination: a useful tool for select patients. Arch Dermatol 2011;147:53–8.

69. DermLite Monitor. 3Gen Inc, San Juan Capistrano (CA). 2015. Available at: http://dermlite.com/products/monitor. Accessed October 7, 2015.

70. Marchetti MA, Fonseca M, Dusza SW, et al. Dermatoscopic imaging of skin lesions by high school students: a cross-sectional pilot study. Dermatol Pract Concept 2015;5:11–28.

71. Janda M, Loescher LJ, Soyer HP. Enhanced skin self-examination: a novel approach to skin cancer monitoring and follow-up. JAMA Dermatol 2013; 149:231–6.

72. Janda M, Loescher LJ, Banan P, et al. Lesion selection by melanoma high-risk consumers during skin self-examination using mobile teledermoscopy. JAMA Dermatol 2014;150:656–8.

73. Manahan MN, Soyer HP, Loescher LJ, et al. A pilot trial of mobile, patient-performed teledermoscopy. Br J Dermatol 2015;172:1072–80.

Index

Dermatol Clin 34 (2016) 363–365
http://dx.doi.org/10.1016/S0733-8635(16)30043-2
0733-8635/16/$ – see front matter

Moving?

Make sure your subscription moves with you!

To notify us of your new address, find your **Clinics Account Number** (located on your mailing label above your name), and contact customer service at:

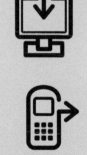

Email: journalscustomerservice-usa@elsevier.com

800-654-2452 (subscribers in the U.S. & Canada)
314-447-8871 (subscribers outside of the U.S. & Canada)

Fax number: 314-447-8029

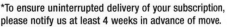

Elsevier Health Sciences Division
Subscription Customer Service
3251 Riverport Lane
Maryland Heights, MO 63043

*To ensure uninterrupted delivery of your subscription, please notify us at least 4 weeks in advance of move.

Printed and bound by CPI Group (UK) Ltd, Croydon, CR0 4YY

17/10/2024

01775515-0001